Ready to Live a High Intensity Life?

Access Free Resources, Bonus Training and Learn Directly From Eric Bakey!

Visit The Website:

www.HighIntensityLife.com

To Read a Personal Letter from Eric Bakey, Author of **Strength From Within**, Flip to the Last Chapter

STRENGTH FROM WITHIN

The Anti-Meathead Approach to Fitness

By Eric Bakey

© 2016 Eric Bakey

All rights reserved.
No portion of this book may be reproduced, stored in a retrieval system, or transmitted in any form or by any means—electronic, mechanical, photocopy, recording, scanning, or other,—except for brief quotations in critical reviews or articles, without the prior written permission of the publisher.

Disclaimer and Terms of Use:
The Author and Publisher has strived to be as accurate and complete as possible in the creation of this book, notwithstanding the fact that he does not warrant or represent at any time that the contents within are accurate due to the rapidly changing nature of the Internet. While all attempts have been made to verify information provided in this publication, the Author and Publisher assumes no responsibility for errors, omissions, or contrary interpretation of the subject matter herein.

Any perceived slights of specific persons, peoples, or organizations are unintentional. In practical advice books, like anything else in life, there are no guarantees of income made. Readers are cautioned to reply on their own judgment about their individual circumstances to act accordingly. This book is not intended for use as a source of legal, medical, health, business, accounting or financial advice. All readers are advised to seek the services of competent professionals in legal, medical, health, business, accounting, and finance fields.

.

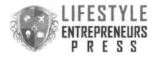

Publisher: Jesse Krieger
Learn More: Jesse@JesseKrieger.com
Get Published: www.LifestyleEntrepreneursPress.com

Lifestyle Entrepreneurs Press
100 Tamal Plaza
Suite 106
Corte Madera, CA 94925

TABLE OF CONTENTS

My Story and Why I Wrote Strength from Within

Despite spending hours in the gym, taking all the supplements GNC will sell you, and reading every fitness article under the sun, do you look pretty much the same as you did last year? I know how frustrating this can be because I've wasted thousands of dollars and an unrecoverable amount of time spinning my wheels in the relentless pursuit of muscle.

Fitness has always been a passion of mine. I wrestled in high school and am a US Army combat veteran who has served with some of the finest in Special Operations in Iraq. Additionally, I'm a Certified Personal Trainer (CPT) through the National Association of Sports Medicine. Still, with a lifetime of both anecdotal and formal health education, I didn't have the physique I saw in all the magazines. The coup de grâce was from a cute girl I was chatting with "down the shore" in Ocean City, Maryland. "You know, you don't look like you work out as much as you do," she observed. There was so much truth in that statement that it hurt like a swift kick to the nuts.

I took myself so seriously and it really hurt to hear, "Do you even lift, bro?" from someone who I hoped appreciated my efforts. I literally hadn't missed a workout in over ten years despite injuries, sicknesses, and deployments. I was often training twice a day, going to the gym five to six days a week, and cramming in yoga, boot camps, and Brazilian Jiu Jitsu anywhere I could. Embarrassingly, I was also dropping around $300 a month on supplements that returned effectively zero for my investment… Not even worth the placebo effect.

Sometimes an outside perspective is what it takes to point out the obvious. I'm eternally grateful for that offhand and humbling comment. That conversation led me down a path where I discovered the importance of diet in supporting physique goals. More importantly, I was able to kick the habitual waste of money that most supplements are as well as apply effective training methods that have stood the test of time.

I debated writing this book for a long time. After making minimal progress for a couple of decades and finally putting the pieces together for myself, I had to ask…

"What do I have to offer?"

Sure, I have achieved such a level of fitness and knowledge in the subject that friends and strangers alike often confide in me for advice. I've worked out in a variety of environments from Gold's Gym to war zone weight piles in battle rattle; from cultish community Crossfit Boxes to solo living room calisthenics. I often joke that fitness isn't hard, and that losing weight is simply a matter of calories in versus calories out. If we simply followed the advice of known experts, we'd all have six-pack abs and be billionaire entrepreneurs.

So what could I write that hasn't already been spelled out explicitly by gurus with PhDs? What can I really say? I stopped writing articles on my blog for a while. Instead I wrote my buddies basic programs that they may or may not have followed. I eventually missed writing and needed a career change from my corporate gig. I took up personal training to give myself the chance to figure out what I wanted to do with the rest of my life. I now get paid to motivate, educate, entertain, and/or bemuse clients in person and in print. It became abundantly clear that I needed to help my clients take a step back from the overwhelming complexity that is the Fitness Industry.

I have often thought about the books and articles I have read about strength training — those from professional bodybuilders, military trainers, and "in the know" fitness experts — and something always seems lacking. Authorities in any field do the basics better than anyone else. But the mastery of the fundamentals allows you to build on your competency and advance to the next stage. This is true for any skill, from learning to speak a language to body shaping!

There is a missing understanding of what mastery of the basics entails until the trainee is elbow deep in the mechanics of it. The technical information seems to be out there, but the art of training and eating right is only partially an academic endeavor. It must be experienced and felt. It's a craft. It is my intention to give you a guide to build the biggest base so that your pyramid of fitness success can grow as high as you'd like to take it. Base building is crucial; and you can build on a strong foundation in fitness and in life. You can take a step back, enjoy "newbie gains" again, and achieve the next level of real fitness!

A Letter to My Twenty-Year-Old Self

Dear Sweet Misguided Eric,

You've been lifting seriously for a while now. You started as a scrawny wrestler, getting smeared by guys with big boulder shoulders, and you wanted to get strong enough not to embarrass yourself on the mat. You developed a decent physique for a natural power-builder, and the super high calorie meals of the United States Army have you bulked up to a soft 235 pounds... not bad for wrestling 152 a few years ago.

I'm writing to you now because you're about to spend thousands of dollars, waste countless hours, and marginalize every relationship you'll have in pursuit of the ever-elusive "perfect body." I'm going to bestow some hard-fought wisdom on you, and although you probably won't listen (don't worry, you're still a hard-headed hard-ass in the future), maybe you'll prevent injury, save money, reach a higher level of fitness, and maybe just enjoy life a little bit more.

I know you're obsessed with "making gains" and you're willing to choke back 300+ grams of protein daily, piss all the colors of the rainbow, and dedicate six to seven days a week driving to Gold's anywhere you are in the world... but I promise, it's not nearly as hard as you're making it. You're still as devoted to training in the future, in fact more than ever, but you're smarter and know how to use laser beam focus to do it right. You're an arrogant, stubborn fool, but I promise if you take my advice now — the earlier the better — you'll reach super-human levels of fitness while the going is good and have a life outside of the gym to boot!

Lifting

I want you to limit yourself to three or four days of training per week. Three is better. I know you're not ready to give up the weights in pursuit of a 315-pound bench press... don't worry, it comes... but you're a sloppy 240 when you get it. When you realize there are guys who weigh less than 180 pounds bench pressing well over 400, you'll be humbled even further. You're never going to be a world-class bench presser, and why would you want to look like one of those guys anyway?

Focus on adding five pounds to the bar every week in a four to six rep range. There is no perfect workout split, so stop program hopping. Get as strong as you can on basic exercises. Muscle follows strength. But be patient, your strength will come. Fight the weight, get one more rep, do or die. You have access to a gym on base, and while it's super convenient, you might as well take advantage. We'll move onto getting REALLY strong for REAL LIFE in a minute.

I guarantee that if you can stop working out all those accessory muscles and focus on what really counts, you'll get bigger and stronger than you ever thought possible. Stop depleting your body's energy recovering from "Arm Day" earlier in the week, and get your incline bench up instead of just pumping the guns.

Lifting weights right now is perfect for you, but since you're in it for the long haul, I'll let you in on a little secret... You don't need heavy weights to get superhuman strong. A weight vest and a kettlebell will be the only equipment you'll need to develop the body of a Greek god.

Do you know how strong you have to be to perform a one arm pull-up? The answer is — very. When you're performing a clean six reps per arm, your back width will widen and your biceps will bulge. Now what happens when you throw on a weight vest or hold a kettlebell? Batwings. It's amazing what happens when you strengthen your body.

I remember looking up at the sky and thinking the first time I was able to complete a set of one-arm push-ups, "Why was I wasting so much time chasing a 345-pound bench when I couldn't even complete one?" Making your body stronger will make your muscles grow. It's really that simple. Don't worry, this secret is safe with us as few other people seemed to have figured it out, "experts" included.

No matter how heavy you go with weighted chins, squats, or presses, you will never get as strong at the bodyweight equivalents. There are progressions that you will have to start at the beginning of regardless of your fitness level, so prepare to be humbled. The fortunate thing is, you can start now, and start anywhere.

This is called The Process. When you focus on the process and the work, everything falls into place. Your strength is a skill, just like any other you need to develop. Training doesn't have to be hard. It should be painful, but brief. Train smarter, not harder.

Health, wealth, relationships, and life purpose are not terribly complicated. But being simple doesn't make them easy. If you actually followed the advice of many of your mentors, you'd have an eight-pack and a billion dollars by the time you're my age... and I'm telling you, while the future is bright... you're not there yet. Don't give up hope. You can do and be anything you want, and you're smart enough to not believe any excuse you give yourself. Never quit, and you'll succeed at whatever you put your mind to.

So when you're ready to start living life instead of living in the gym, learn the bodyweight progressions. At least don't spend your vacations seeking out Big Box Gyms, or every day of the week driving across town to pump your ego. There is a better way.

Don't neglect stretching or some brief cardio. You need to cut weight before you will be able to make any progress on the bodyweight stuff, so focus on brisk walking on your off days until you build the cardio to go for a few miles of running. The army demands that you run two miles every six months, but you know you can do better than that. (Disclaimer, you eventually work to a sub 11:00 two-mile run, you PT stud you.)

Now when you get deployed, if you're still stuck using weights, you're going to cut your training back to two days a week. You're not sleeping, going on long missions, and burning a ton of calories... There is no need to give up ALL your hard-fought muscle. Your Iraq weight-pile workouts will look like this:

Monday
Squat
Bench Press
Assistance work

Thursday
Deadlift
Press
Assistance work

You're on patrol, running, shooting-moving-communicating, and all around very stressed out seven days a week. Focus on maintaining what you've got, but you'll be surprised how strong you'll get when you train smart and train with purpose.

Eating

Don't get strong and fat or skinny and weak. The reality is you have to build muscle in order to burn the fat and reveal it. The truth is you don't need a ton of supplements or 5,000 calories a day to get bigger. When you starve yourself on top of running to lose fat, you end up burning off hard-earned muscle. Your body doesn't like to cooperate, so here is the cheat sheet:

Eat three meals per day to gain muscle. Two if you're getting fat.

Before you work out (fasted) drink half a scoop of protein powder for the BCAAs to maintain muscle mass.

After you work out, eat your carbs, at least 50% of your daily carbohydrates should come in the meal after you work out. *Spoiler alert, there is no "anabolic window" and you need to consume real food, not just "BRO-tein" shakes.

Roadwork

The Fresh Prince of Bel-Air turns out to be a pretty smart guy... to paraphrase, he said If you want to be successful, you need to do two things. You need to read and you need to run.

Get your roadwork in the morning, on an empty stomach. Listen to podcasts or books on tape. That Tony Robbins audiobook will eventually change your life, so the earlier the better.

Run. Sprints suck, but do them anyway. Sprint hills. You don't need to do them every day, but if you can't move your body, you're dead. Iraq shows you this.

You'll never be the biggest or the fastest person in the world, but you can put in the work to be the best version of yourself. Sprints are more humbling than insults or failing at a bench press attempt.

Don't forget to stretch after your runs. You want to be refreshed and limber for your bodyweight moves. They will keep you agile and flexible, so don't worry about becoming a bendy yoga weirdo.

Life

Look into Stoic philosophy sooner than later. Remember roadwork and audio books? Don't stress about the future or the past. You can't time travel, read minds, or change things that are not in your control. You can control your feelings when things happen to you that are out of your control. Be present, seek to master your emotional state, and therefore master yourself. Work The Process.

Your mind is a muscle that needs to be trained just as hard as (if not harder than) your biceps. Developing mental resilience takes time, and it's a skill that you need to work to develop, just like being able to do a handstand. Don't get frustrated because your goals seem too far away. You can do it if you put in the work.

Read more. Stand on the shoulders of giants. Since you're painfully introverted (still) you can use books as mentors and get the cheat sheet for life.

Train more. The more frequently you can recover from your training, the more you can train. It doesn't work vice versa.

Your mind expands when you read. Just don't get too lost in it...

No matter how articulate the author, you need to DO if you want to BE.

You grow and become stronger in many ways when you train. You must overcome the physical pain and demand that your muscles provide you the ability to do what was impossible the week before. You force yourself to endure despite adversity in an attempt to defy gravity and your genes.

Your mind and body go hand in hand. Never stop moving forward, no matter how slow the pace. Progress is progress. Having a growth mind-set and a positive mental attitude is the key to both genius and the physique of your dreams. Focus is a skill that you need to develop. It will help you overcome the fear of missing out. Take care of your mind and body by making time for self-care, and your business will take care of itself.

And most of all, the quality of your life is the quality of your relationships. Do not try to go it alone... You'll learn that you can have anything you want in this life if you're willing to help enough other people get what they want. Clarity will come from taking action, and you're going to mess up plenty in the process. However, the sooner you can embrace empathy, honest humility, and open up to some uncomfortable vulnerability, you'll get the feedback you need to become an outstanding leader.

Love,
Your future self

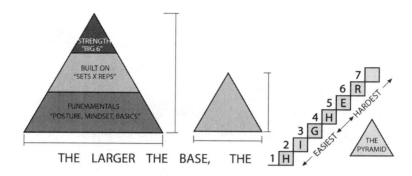

The Pyramid

High-tech machines and periodization programs haven't changed the basics of training or gravity... Man has pursued a superior physique for millennia! The modern era of bodybuilding is approaching the century mark. So how do you get there? Get strong at the basic human movements, and use your own body weight before you ever drive across town to set foot in a commercial gym again.

Why So Much Confusion?

The problem is not a lack of information available about the subject; there is simply too much of it. There is so much conflicting advice out there and the complexity leads to distraction. It should be noted that complication is the enemy of progress. The purpose of this book is to simplify and dispel some popular myths that I, too, believed for a long time to the detriment of progress. When it comes to physique change, the magic happens when you eliminate distraction and focus on Keeping It Stupid-Simple.

This book is also about self mastery. Use this book with cautious excitement. I hope to instill a burning desire to cast aside the unnecessary, to spend as little time in the purgatory of uncertainty, and to create lasting habit change — right now.

Over 70% of people, when given the simple instruction by their doctors to take up a walking habit to slow down or reverse the debilitating effects of heart disease, take no action. Such a simple prescription that could save their lives and drastically increase the quality prefer to take no steps, literally, to abate their demise. To me this is tragic, absurd, and I wouldn't imagine the audience reading this book would ever find themselves in such a condition. However, if you want to gain the most from this book, you need to set and accomplish "micro-goals."

The studies show — as well as my anecdotal experience proves — the urgency of now. This book will lay out a process to achieve an elite level of fitness. It may very well be the last training book you ever need, but unless you take action right this second… the chances are, you will never complete this book or create lasting change in your life toward accomplishing your fitness goals. Stop right now and do just one push-up.

Seriously.

Just one.

There is power of taking just one small step in the right direction toward any goal.

Put the book down. Put your hands on the floor. Slowly lower your chest to the ground, and then push yourself away from the gravity of Earth.

Did you do it?

No one is watching. It's just you, me, and your mind… you'll do thousands of push-ups in your life, but you have the opportunity to remember this first one. This first rep toward accomplishing your goal of self-mastery means something. Do you have the courage to take on this challenge? In knowing one thing, you know ten thousand. Know thyself.

Do one. Just one. It's the first step on a long journey that begins right now.

"Would you have a great empire? Rule over yourself." ~Publilius Syrus

Don't turn another page until you do ONE push-up.

Strength from Within

22

A Different Approach

"When you find yourself on the side of the majority, it's time to stop and think." ~Mark Twain

How do two extremely satisfying meals a day, complemented by three days a week of basic strength training exercises that you can perform anywhere sound? It is in total contrast to what is pushed by the "heath and fitness" comics as well as the supplement companies. I would also bet that it sounds different and more refreshing than the approach you're currently following.

In this book, I will outline a logical, sustainable, and proven method to achieve your fitness goals that will change your physique as well as your view of the fitness industry as a whole. Fitness is something that should enhance our lives but not be the focus of it. Consistency is key in any skill, and you owe it to yourself to set yourself free from the lies and lack of progress. Finally, real world strength and a jaw-dropping physique is something anyone who's willing to put in the work can accomplish. Achieving expert level strength is simple in its execution, but it is not easy.

I've read old gymnastic tomes, viewed the modern scientific studies, drawn from the bodybuilding methods before steroids, tested these methods on hundreds of clients, and personally achieved elite levels of fitness. This program is the culmination of over ten years of applicable trial and error, and the same one I use to coach my personal training clients to achieve the body of their dreams all over the world.

Less is more in my approach:

1. Focus on diet for recovery and training for strength in real life.

For long-term success, both diet and training are of critical importance. However, if you've been struggling with your muscle growth or fat loss goals, you've likely been emphasizing the wrong components of physique change. Looking to gain muscle? Getting really strong at basic movements should be your priority as that is what will drive muscular adaptations. Your nutrition is what will allow you to recover and grow, given the right training stimulus. Looking to lose fat? Your nutrition is set up to permit muscle retention while letting the food you eat drive the change in your body composition. The Holy Grail is when you're looking to build muscle and loose fat. It's certainly possible when both your diet and your training are in sync.

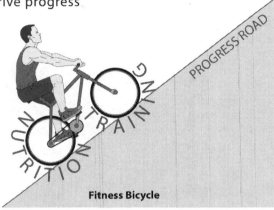

Nutrition and training as two wheels that drive progress

PROGRESS ROAD

TRAINING

NUTRITION

Fitness Bicycle

2. Simplify things as much as possible.

Training to get strong with your body weight before you ever touch a barbell is a crucial step in the fitness journey. Get everything you can out of all that you've got before seeking answers elsewhere. There are six key gymnastic movements that will allow you to make the most profound strength and physique changes. Master these basic human movements, and you will have the body of a Greek god, and the athleticism to excel through any challenge. In regard to diet, a reduced meal frequency makes it possible to eat bigger, more satisfying meals, and yet still feel full while losing weight. This is possible whether you are cutting or bulking, and it simplifies your life immensely.

How the Body Moves, the Mind Grooves:
A Primer on Posture and Growth Mind-Set

Your health and mind-set are not fixed. You are in control of both. Not your genes, not your friends, not your environment, but you. Developing a growth mind-set for health can be difficult if you've spent your entire life thinking with a fixed mind-set.

Everyone has their own definition of "healthy." Losing fat, eating nutritious food, building muscle, and sleeping enough are the modalities I use in my personal definition and pursuit. Developing a growth mind-set to health will allow you to define it for yourself, focus on the process, and not solely rely on the results of your practice. You are the result of the habits you've had up to this point. If you choose better habits, you will be able to accomplish what others who've come before you have accomplished. Failure is only one instance; it is not a person.

In failure we achieve growth in our lives, but especially in the pursuit of muscle.

First, you have to decide that health is a priority and how you are going to define it. You need to know what you want to achieve and focus on setting yourself up for success. If you want to lose fat, don't focus on your "ideal weight." Instead, commit to exercising consistently and making better food choices. If you wanted to wake up with the energy required to crush it in life and unleash epic power, make sleep a priority and enforce your bedtime.

Notice and acknowledge the little voice in the back of your head when you feel the resistance to change. When you start exercising or cooking healthier, you may hear, "You can't do this. You were born this way!" That's your fixed mind-set pitting your cognitive distortions against you. Your growth mind-set will allow you to know that the pain is temporary, that it gets easier every day, and you can do it if you focus on easy wins. The mind is quick to justify feelings, and it often does so incorrectly. These false realities are delusions, and in reality, small progress is still progress. Focus on getting 1% better, every day.

Be aware of your emotions and choose to focus on the positive ones that you feel when you accomplish small victories. You must recognize the wins in order to build upon them. Emotional states lead you to taking action, and taking action is what gets us what we want. We want to build stronger, leaner, bodies, but it all starts with a positive mind-set. Therefore, bulging deltoids are as much the result of working our shoulders as they are strengthening feelings of happy emotions when we choose to focus on our positive self-image.

Even if you do slip up, realize that failure is what provides the conduit to growth. Failure is not a reason to give up. Everyone experiences failure, and the heroes we celebrate have failed more than you've ever tried. They continue to get back to it and put in the hard work. That is what makes them stand out. Recognize what is keeping you from your success. If you couldn't go to bed early enough to get restful sleep, think about what prevented it… Maybe don't watch TV in the evening? Show up again the next day, and try again. You may have failed to get your workout in today, it's not a reason to give up on your whole routine. Make an "at least" list. You may not have the energy for a full workout, but you can at least do a few push-ups or jumping jacks. At least get your heart pumping for a few minutes. The things you can accomplish if you focus on getting "at least" a few things done might be all the mind-set shift you need to accomplish your bigger goal. You can always try again tomorrow, but at least do something with the time you've got today.

You must show up consistently. When you do, big results will happen. However, you must focus on the process of growth, not the end result. Instead of thinking about how much weight you have to lose or how big you want your muscles to be, focus on consistently eating healthy and intelligent training. Trust in the process, believe in yourself, and fitness will become effortless.

Finally, you must take responsibility for where you are currently. You cannot make progress when you live with excuses. If you cannot accept that statement, you should probably just quit reading. Stop using money as an excuse to not eat healthy or being too busy as an excuse not to get enough sleep. I'm sure you've spent money and time on things that did not prioritize your health. Instead of saying, "I don't have time to eat quality food or go to bed on time." Realize what you're saying is that you don't want to prioritize your health. Can you hear me now?

Take responsibility for your health in the state it is in now. Your mind-set must not be that of the "victim" of poor genes or a busy schedule. Students must earn their grades, and so must you earn the body of your dreams. When you do, you get to enjoy your hard work so much more. Musicians tune their instruments, carpenters sharpen their saws, and athletes train their bodies. So must you do the work to unveil the body of your dreams.

Habits, both good and bad must be trained. In order to make the good habits stick, we must acknowledge what they are and build upon them. To change a bad habit, we must acknowledge it as well and seek to fulfill the need that is detracting from our goal by redirecting. Feed the need, not the craving, with more positive habits. This switch can be achieved by focusing on foundational habits and small wins. A foundational habit provides the launch pad for all the rest of your daily small wins. They are the habits that position you for easy successes and build exponential confidence. Accomplishing foundational habits helps you achieve your daily goals as well as create a cascade of positive changes that allow you to accomplish more than you ever thought possible.

Before we get into the intense training section, I wanted to get you started on the right foot on your complete physical and mental transformation. Your brain is an organ, and your "mental muscle" is a function that needs to be trained just as hard, if not harder, than your biceps. Your most concrete interaction with the world is through your body, but your nervous system constantly receives information from both the environment and your inner dialogue. Why do we say, "I think…" but not, "I am my expanding and contracting my lungs"? We can affect our entire system by tinkering with our mind-set through movement and posture. Through conscious thought alone, it would be difficult to not be affected by fear, anger, or a host of other emotions. You can give your mind a break by focusing on the fundamentals that allow for incredible mental fortitude.

Instead of going through the day in a reactive state to the plethora of information being tweeted, notified, and friend requested to you, you have the power to not only hold a strong defense to these distractions but apply a strategic offense to combat them as well. Your entire reality is filtered through the nervous system. A positive mind-set and strong posture have the ability to make you physically sturdy, emotionally resilient, and give you the energy to live life to the fullest. These deceptively simple tools enable progress in all aspects of your life. Many books have been written on the power of a positive mental attitude and meditation practices. Instead of writing another on these subjects, I will encourage you to put "body checks" and posture exercises into your fitness practice. Good posture not only dictates how the world sees you but, better yet, short circuits any negative self-talk and defeatist language you may be communicating within yourself. The brain physically changes based on how we move.

It should be no surprise to you that sitting at your computer all day will make a mess of your spine, leave your postural muscles weak, and sap you of the energy required to perform at your best. Even recent trends of stability balls as chairs and standing desks do little to prevent an impending hunchback. Ensuring you engage your posture muscles and maintain a more erect spinal alignment will become easier with consistent training. Use external cues such as a timer or cue yourself with silly, self-imposed rules. For example, every time you walk through a doorway, you must take a few seconds to correct your posture. Do this multiple times per day.

You are always training your body. Every time you do something, it is re-enforced in the brain whether you like it or not, so choose better habits to train. An unchecked, poor posture has the potential to last a lifetime. Ensure you train your body to sit, stand, and lift heavy objects properly to avoid negative repercussions in both short-term and future health. Poor posture indicates a lack of strength and control of the upper body, which leads to inadequate flexibility and increased stress on the body's systems. Undue stress while sitting or standing affects energy output because poor posture forces all of your internal organs down causing your belly to protrude. Standing upright in the correct position will help promote a smooth flow through the gastrointestinal tract, make you look leaner, and give you more energy. When sitting, make sure you keep both feet planted firmly on the ground and distribute your weight evenly. Crossing your legs cuts off circulation and puts uneven pressure on your vertebrae. Whenever you're sitting, standing, or walking do not allow your chin to jut forward. Keep your head in alignment with your shoulders to avoid "text neck."

Do you ever find yourself looking down at the ground, or off into the distance when confronted by challenging people? Do you ever find that you're holding your breath when you face difficult circumstances? Do you have nervous ticks (foot tapping, nail biting, etc.) when in a stressful situation? These are just a few of the obvious symptoms of not adequately performing body checks and, chances are, your posture is reflecting your threatened internal state.

Think of your mind-set as a filter through which you receive and process new information from the environment. A negative mind-set causes blockages in your "world-view filter" and is commonly, and visibly, reflected in one or more of your physical traits. Examples are: poor posture, eyebrow furrowing, jaw clenching, raised shoulders, rounded upper back, a sunken chest, belly tension, hips held back (anterior tilt), or held forward (posterior tilt). All of these are indications that you are not fully present with your body and often accompanied by shallow breathing. None of these are a good look and certainly not indicative of a confident, positive individual.

You will find that by correcting your posture, restoring breathing mechanics, and focusing on a positive growth mind-set, you will not only feel better but also you will LOOK better.

Many people have a misconception as to what "good posture" is. Often they thrust out their chest and retract the shoulders in an exaggerated manner while arching their lower back. Good posture should hold the head balanced and erect, chest high without tension, abdomen flat, shoulders back and relaxed, and lower back only slightly curved. Surprisingly, good posture is not second nature to most people and in fact, many feel more natural maintaining a poor posture. But don't worry, holding good posture can be learned and is easily attainable. Specific muscles need to be trained in order to maintain good posture without undue fatigue. Here are my five favorite exercises for strengthening postural muscles, and in return, setting your mind right for peak performance in any athletic or social event. Perform them as an energizer any time of day!

EXERCISE 1:
1. Swing arms forward and upward to full stretch overhead and at the same time rise high on toes.
2. Swing arms sideward and downward slowly and press back hard. At the same time retract chin and let heels drop to the ground. Avoid an exaggerated arch in lower back. Perform 10 repetitions.

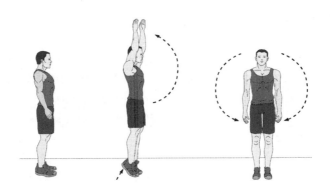

Chi-Y Raise

EXERCISE 2:
1. Torso leaning forward about 60°, arms hanging downward loosely from shoulders.
2. Swing arms sideward and backward vigorously, retracting

chin forcefully and flattening upper back. Hold this contracted position for a hard two-count and perform 10 repetitions.

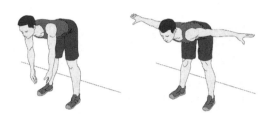

Bent Lateral Raise

EXERCISE 3:

1. Leaning slightly forward, elbows bent, and fingertips touching shoulders.
2. Make small circles about a foot in diameter, elbows circling upward and backward. Press arms backward and retract head. Movement is slow. Perform 10 repetitions forward and 10 backward.

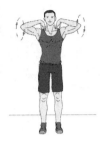

Bent Arm Circles

EXERCISE 4:

1. Leaning slightly forward, arms horizontally at sides, palms up.
2. Make small circles about a foot in diameter, hands circling upward and backward. Press arms backward and retract head in line with shoulders. Movement is slow. Perform 10 repetitions forward and 10 backward.

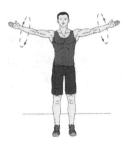

Large Arm Circles

EXERCISE 5:

1. Start with your arms overhead.
2. Pull arms slowly downward until fists are beside shoulders. Pull as though doing a behind-the-neck pull-up. Squeeze rhomboid muscles tight as if crushing a pencil between your shoulder blades. Hold this contracted position for a hard two-count, and perform 10 repetitions.

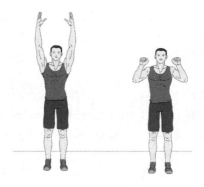

Behind the Neck Pulldown

EXERCISE 6:

1. (1) Back against the wall
2. (2) With your tongue on the roof of your mouth, force your neck straight, and retract into a double chin. Hold this unattractive position for a three-count, and perform 10 repetitions.

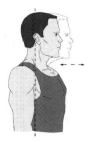

Double Chin Posture Exercise

You can do these as energizers any time of the day, and better yet, multiple times a day. Perform these exercises and you will be well on your way to approaching life with a more positive attitude and stance. You will perform better in all areas of your life when your inward state is reflected in your outward posture, as well as be able to short circuit negative beliefs when you stand comfortably tall and confident.

Crash Course in the Components of Fitness

Muscular Strength

"Strong people are harder to kill
and more useful in general."
~ Mark Rippetoe

The basic concept of progressive overload has been understood for thousands of years. Muscles increase in size and strength with regular and continually challenging exercise. They grow weaker when not trained, and thus, use it or lose it. Strength is best developed in muscles when they contract through maximum loads. Strenuous callisthenic exercises, resistance training, and sprinting are excellent strength-developing activities. Muscle follows strength; you must get stronger in order to build muscle.

Cardio-Respiratory Endurance

Rather than seeking the massive bodybuilder type look, we are aiming to achieve an athletic gymnastic build that is as much "Go" as it is "Show." This requires a certain level of conditioning in order to access all the benefits of a lean athletic physique. Developing endurance permits an individual to continue strenuous activity for many hours without fatigue and gives them the ability to go the distance! Being in shape is characterized by a greater than average amount of muscular strength and a level of cardiovascular fitness to move! You must continue to challenge your internal network to make it possible for the blood to deliver increased amounts of oxygen and nutrition to your muscles. Equally as important, your blood stream carries away waste products that would leave your muscles cramped and immobile. The kinds of exercise needed to build up muscular endurance are the same as those needed for strength training. As a bonus, cardio increases the efficiency of your muscles as well as the overall functioning of the heart, vascular system, and lungs. It should be noted that running is not the only way to develop cardio-respiratory endurance!

Body Composition

Everyone is born with a six-pack of abs and we aim to keep a low level of body fat in order to showcase those strong functional muscles. In addition to having a lower body fat level for aesthetics, you will be pound-for-pound stronger to complete more difficult strength feats. Simply put, it is easier to do more pull-ups when you weigh less! Lean muscle mass is what we are after, and it is key to mastering your bodyweight movements.

Flexibility & Agility

Being flexible is crucial in the development of coordination and in injury prevention. It integrates all parts of the body into efficient, purposeful effort. Agility is being able to change direction and the position of the body with great speed. It enables you fall to the ground without injury or leap to your feet quickly. Conditioning exercises that require extensive and rapid changes of position like competitive sports, as well as athletic drills, best develop this important component of physical fitness. Superfluous movements are eliminated, energy is conserved, and endurance is increased when you are a flexible and agile athlete.

How a Minimalist Approach Incorporates All the Components

In case it hasn't been made clear yet, we are after the lean-mean-athletic gymnast look that women love and guys envy. I will lay out a plan to achieve this physique that you can take with you anywhere and is infinitely scalable. I developed this plan out of both necessity and desperation. I've spent over fifteen years experimenting, researching, and applying the principles I will outline for you now.

The beauty of this approach is that you do not need to perform these exercises in a traditional gym. You can continue to progress on the Key Movements, perform posture exercises, and focus on what really gets you the physique you desire no matter your zip code. Looking back, it really is as simple as getting stronger on a few exercises and scaling them for your individual strength levels that will yield the results you desire. Hindsight is not always 20/20, but I've connected the dots between taking muscles to real muscular failure, failure's effect on muscular development, and being able to train anywhere to achieve your goals.

Before you set out on one more expedition to the gym, and pay one more month's dues consider the value of your own body versus gravity. Why lay down under a perfectly balanced iron bar for a bench press when you can't do ten perfectly executed one-arm incline push-ups? Think about the transfer of strength and growth that this will have on your physique. Take a break from your normal bodybuilding magazine "bro split" designed to keep you buying, not progressing.

MASTER the basics, and reap new rewards when you're able to overcome the world's gravitational pull on your own body in planes of motion that will develop a functional and aesthetically pleasing build. No longer will you "pick things up and put them down" in the same way. IF you do go back to the gym, you will be leaner, stronger, and more athletic than ever before. So take a break with me, leave the latest Mr. Olympia arms routine alone, and let's get really strong!

Getting Strong for Real Life:
Anywhere, Any Time.

You do not need any fancy equipment to get the body of your dreams. Sculpting your muscles using bodyweight movements is the ideal way to develop a truly powerful physique. Most gymnasts, from the high school level all the way up to Olympic champions, have ridiculously muscular bodies. Success leaves clues. Training for power is optimal and calisthenics are king. Stick to the fundamentals, focusing on a movement practice that unleashes your muscles' true strength rather than just "working out." Having a plan of attack to achieve success in fitness, nutrition, and ultimately life that is centered around simplicity is the best way to reach your goals in the least amount of time.

You do not need access to a gym to develop muscles that will give you the body of a Greek god. No commuting, no waiting for equipment, and no excuses. The beauty of bodyweight workouts is that you can perform them anywhere and anytime. It is preferable to use your body weight because the strength you gain is entirely functional and athletic. Taking a step back and focusing on getting everything you can out of all you've got will take you to a level of fitness that rivals (and in my opinion is superior) to the most diehard of gym rats. I will lay out key exercises that you should pursue mastery in to gain the maximum benefit to your physique.

Even the strongest gymnasts cannot perform all these exercises with perfect form, and in that vein these exercises are infinitely scalable. I challenge you to control your body weight in these exercises before you crank out one more set of traditional "Pumping Iron" bicep curls. Your success performing these exercises will have the greatest carryover to real life and will demand respect from fellow athletes as well as admiration from the opposite sex.

Mastering the following "Big Six" bodyweight exercises should be your focus, and I will suggest a number of different routines that will optimize your progress. Achieving muscular failure under mechanical disadvantage is what allows us to develop muscle using only our body weight. That being said, it would be foolish to climb under 500 pounds and try to squat the weight if you had not laid down the foundational strength required to do such a task. We must build a strong foundation of muscular strength, flexibility, and general fitness of our entire system if we ever hope to accomplish these athletic feats of strength.

Prior to switching to bodyweight strength training, I was able to bench press 345 pounds, squat 455 pounds, and deadlift 515 pounds at a body weight of 189. While these numbers are moderately impressive for gym-rats, no one ever asked me outside of a gym how much I benched unless I cued them in on my dedication to fitness. It was quite frustrating due to how much effort I put into accomplishing these numbers and the toll it took on my body and social life. I spent six days a week tied to a gym membership, would panic when thinking about missing workouts due to travel, and incurred injuries regularly while grunting under iron. All of my fitness problems were solved, and I was able to live a more social life, with bodyweight training! Now, my sleeves bulge with functional muscle while working out in the park and people ask me how much I bench. I think back to those endless years driving to a dark, dingy gym, smile, and say I don't.

Executing the Big Six movements for multiple repetitions, in our case for truly strong individuals, are the equivalent to elite level lifts. Trying to skip steps in order to accomplish the movements will more often than not cause injury and halt progress. Work your way through the progressions to build a strong foundation for reaching new heights in fitness. Remember the Fitness Pyramid — the wider the base, the higher level of strength you can reach. Your tendons and ligaments need time to grow to keep up with your muscles. If you try to progress too quickly, you may cause an injury, and you will certainly plateau well before you've gotten the most benefit from climbing the progress latter rung by rung.

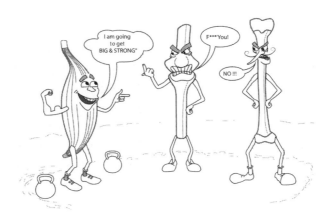

Tendons, Ligaments, Joints vs. Muscles Cartoon

1. Handstand Push-up

Forget about overhead presses, and look no further than the handstand push-up for the ultimate shoulder builder. Someone who can military press his body weight with a barbell is considered very strong. When you can use a full range of motion for multiple reps using only your body weight, your shoulders will pop with functional strength. The handstand push-up requires the ability to keep your core tight while holding yourself upside-down on your hands. To perform the handstand push-up, assume a handstand position. Slowly bend your elbows and lower your inverted body toward the ground. In order to maintain balance, you're going to have to call on your core and other smaller stabilizing muscles. If you can't do a stand-alone handstand, use a wall to assist you. Once you can do a handstand push-up on the flat ground, you can add a level of difficulty by extending the range of motion by placing your hands on phonebooks, bricks, or those fancy push-up handles.

Handstand push-ups can easily be regressed by changing the leverage. If you aren't able to do a full handstand push-up, start with a pike push-up by putting your feet up on a chair or step and bending your body at the waist. This places less of your weight in your arms while still strengthening your shoulders.

Handstand push-ups against the wall are great, but the freestanding handstand push-up is the next step. Performing a freestanding handstand push-up requires incredible athleticism, stability, and strength to lower all the way down and press yourself back up. To gain the ultimate in bodyweight mastery, I challenge you to pursue the one-arm handstand push-up! You've got yourself a serious challenge that can take years to master and requires no gym membership whatsoever.

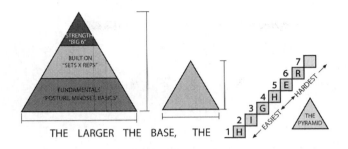

THE LARGER THE BASE, THE

Use The Pyramid

Progression:

Step I - Incline Pike Push-up 3x30
Step II - Pike Push-up 3x30
Step III - Pike Push-up Diamond 2x20
Step IIII - Decline Pike Diamond Push-up 2x20
Step V - Wall Headstands 2min
Step VI - Crow Stand 1min
Step VII - Wall Handstand 2min
Step VIII - Half Handstand Push-up 2x20
Step IIX - Handstand Push-up 2x15
Step IX - Close Handstand Push-up 2x12
Step X - Uneven Handstand Push-up 2x10
Step XI - 1/2 One-Arm Handstand Push 2x8
Step XII - Lever Handstand Push-up 2x6
Bodyweight Master Level - One-Arm Handstand Push-up 2x5

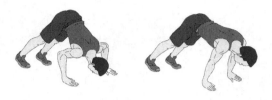

Beginner: Pike Pushup

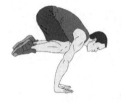

Intermediate: Crow Stand

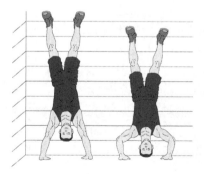

Advanced: Handstand Pushup

2. One-Arm Pull-Up

There are few better examples of pound-for-pound strength that will provide a host of physique building benefits than the one-arm pull-up. Though a solid foundation in two-arm pull-ups is a prerequisite for performing this move, the one-arm pull-up is an exercise that requires lots of patience and training to perform.

Pull-ups are a highly effective exercise that works a whole host of muscle groups, not just your back. Your biceps will bulge with functional strength when you can perform multiple reps of one-arm pull-ups. As with all bodyweight exercises, they can be performed anywhere.

If you don't have access to a proper pull-up bar, monkey bars or even a tree limb at a park, you can throw a towel over a sturdy door and perform strict pull-ups that will increase your back width as well as forearm strength.

Progression:
Dead hang 1min
Jackknife Pull-up 3x20
Half Pull-up 2x15
Full Pull-up 2x10
Close Pull-up 2x10
Uneven Pull-up 2x9
1/2 One-Arm Pull-up 2x8
Assisted One-Arm Pull-up 2x7
Assisted Negative One-Arm 2x7
One-Arm Pull-up 2x6

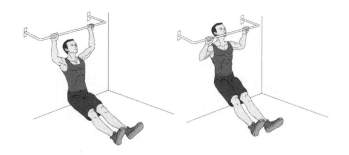

Beginner: Jackknife Pull

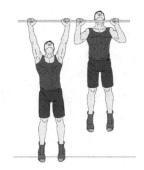

Intermediate: Full Pull-up

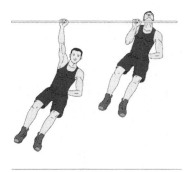

Advanced: One-Arm Pull-up

3. Pistol Squat

The ability to squat a lot of weight with two legs can be impressive, but even those who can barbell squat twice their body weight often struggle with the strength, stability, and flexibility needed to do a pistol. Though the pistol is a leg exercise, it demands full body strength and more athleticism than the traditional barbell squat. Avid lifters are often caught off guard the first time they try this move, so be prepared to be humbled by its deceptively simple performance. Just like the other moves on this list, you can work toward doing pistol squats by changing the leverage or giving yourself an assist from an external object. Once you've developed the strength to perform multiple repetitions, you can advance the exercise by adding speed, jumps, or even some external weight in your hands.

The pistol squat requires strength building of the quads, hamstrings, glutes, hips, and inner thighs. These muscles can be developed utilizing the traditional prisoner squat. Place your hands behind your head, squat down until your thighs are below parallel. Make sure you squeeze your glutes as you come up.

You can advance this exercise by adding weight held over your head or building speed. Build explosive power by performing squat jumps and advanced variations of one legged squats affectionately called shrimps!

Progression:
Jackknife Squat 3x40
Supported Squat 3x30
Half Squat 2x50
Full Squat 2x30
Close Squat 2x20
Uneven Squat 2x20
Bulgarian Split Squat 2x20
Box Squat 2x20
Half One-Leg Squat 2x20
Assisted One-Leg Squat 2x20

Pistol Squat 2x20
Renegade Pistol 2x20
Intermediate Shrimp 2x20
Full Shrimp 2x20
Elevated Shrimp 2x20

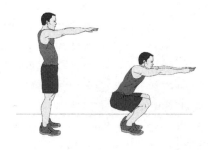

Beginner: Full Squat

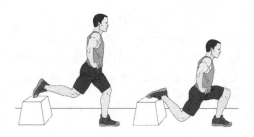

Intermediate: Bulgarian Split Squat

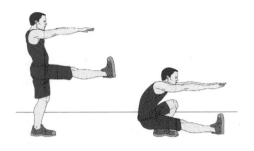

Advanced: Pistol Squat

4. Muscle-Up

Muscle-ups combine the classic pull-up and dip along with the addition of the deceptively difficult transition phase. In my opinion, this is the Holy Grail of upper body exercises. Besides developing a visually pleasing and functional upper-body, the muscle-up also requires tremendous abdominal recruitment. Even being able to do double-digit repetitions of pull-ups and dips, it can still take a considerable amount of practice and strength to perform even one muscle-up. A note for those hardcore, never-leave-the-house, home-gym types who only have a doorway pull-up bar — you are going to have to go outside to practice the final stages after you gain a baseline of strength. You will be rewarded with newfound muscle and athleticism.

Progression:
Step 1: Horizontal Row
Step 2: Incline Row
Step 3: Ring Pull-up
Step 4: False Grip Pull-up
Step 5: Push-up
Step 6: Decline Push-up
Step 7: Assisted Dip
Step 8: Ring Dip

Step 9: Jumping Muscle-up

Step 10: Negative Muscle-up

Step 11: Assisted Muscle-up

Step 12: Kipping Muscle-up

Step 13: Full Muscle-up

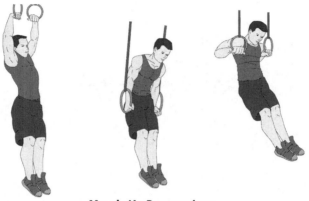

Muscle Up Progressions

5. One-Hand Push-up

"How much ya bench?" is the typical question asked of anyone who's involved in fitness. I've seen people who can bench press over 300 pounds not have the strength to perform one-handed push-ups, myself included. When you can perform one-handed push-ups with ease, make it more difficult by placing your feet on a chair. You'll develop a fantastic boxy upper chest that looks great and performs even better. You don't need a spotter to perform them, so you can actually achieve true muscular failure without fear of strangling yourself with a traditional bench press. One-handed push-ups are an awesome way to develop a champion chest!

Developing the strength to perform the one handed push-up requires strengthening multiple muscle groups including the chest, shoulders, triceps and an extremely rigid core. And the great thing about it is that the exercise can be easily modified to increase difficultly and work different muscle groups. Adjusting the placement of your hands narrower and wider will emphasize different muscle groups. The narrower your hand placement, the more you will target the triceps, while a wider hand placement emphasizes your pecs.

Progression:
Wall Push-up 3x50
Incline Push-up 3x40
Kneeling Push-up 3x30
Half Push-up 2x25
Full Push-up 2x20
Diamond Push-up 2x20
Decline Diamond Push-up 2x20
Uneven Push-up 2x20
Lever Push-up 2x20
Incline One-Arm Push-up 2x20
Half One-Arm Push-up 2x20
One-Arm Push-up 2x10
Decline One-Arm Push-up 2x5

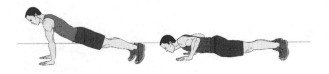

Beginner: Pushup

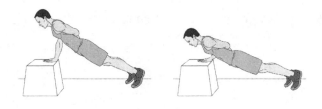

Intermediate: Incline-One Arm Pushup

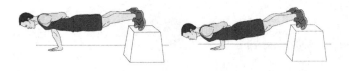

Advanced: Decline One-Arm Pushup

6. L-Sit

The L-sit is a fundamental gymnastic isometric exercise that requires holding your body upright on your palms with your legs held straight out so the shape of your body resembles a capital letter "L."

This emphasizes the abs, but it really works your entire body. You'll also need powerful triceps and better than average flexibility in your hips and hamstrings to hold this position.

Start by mastering the Hanging Leg Raise.

Progression:
Knee Tuck 3x40
Flat Knee Raise 3x35
Flat Bent Leg Raise 3x30
Flat Frog Raise 3x25
Flat Straight Leg Raise 2x20
Hanging Knee Raise 2x15
Hanging Bent-Leg Raise 2x15
Hanging Frog Raise 2x15
Partial Straight Leg Raise 2x15
Hanging Straight Leg Raise 2x30
Hanging Bent Leg V-Raise 2x15
Hanging Straight Leg V-Raise 2x30
Hanging Toes to Bar 2x30
Hanging V-Raise Windshield Wipers 2x15
Ice cream Maker 2x15
One-Arm Hanging Leg Raise 2x30

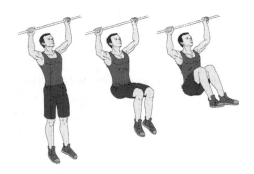

Beginner: Hanging Knee Raise

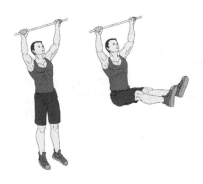

Intermediate: Hanging Straight-leg V-Raise

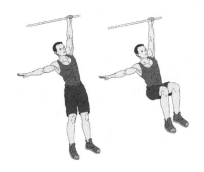

Advanced: One-Arm Hanging Leg Raise

As with all of these exercises, scaling to your current fitness level is easy. The first version is with the knees down. Start on all fours with your hands shoulder width apart and at eye level. Keeping your arms straight, walk your hands forward as far as you can. Don't let your hips and stomach sag as you walk your hands out. If you can reach the fully outstretched position, your stomach should not be touching the floor. Walk your hands back to the starting position. That's one rep. Once you can perform ten reps with your knees down, you're ready for the advanced version where you'll start in a push-up position with your knees up and legs straight.

Progression:

Step 1: Foot Supported L-Sit Hold - 1 minute

Step 2: Tucked L-Sit - 1 Minute

Step 3: Straddle L-Sit - 70 Seconds

Step 4: V Sit - 2x20 Seconds

Step 5: *Master Level* L-Sit - 60 seconds

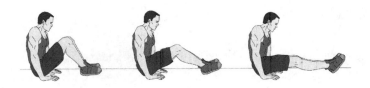

Beginner: Tucked L-Sit

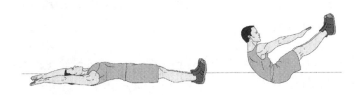

Intermediate: V-Sit

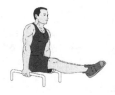

Advanced: L-Sit

Bonus Back Bridge

The bridge requires a degree of mobility that can be challenging for a lot of strong people. Even if you do not wish to give up your beloved weights, practicing toward a full back bridge can be a great way to improve mobility in your shoulders, pelvis, and spine. It strengthens all the muscles used while performing the deadlift, and can be used as a warm-up or finisher to your workout. From strengthening your glutes, spinal erectors, and other posterior musculature to providing a stretch for your hip flexors, abs, shoulders and chest, the benefits of bridging are a very healthy addition to a well-rounded strength training program.

Even if you decide to keep your traditional strength training regiment utilizing traditional weight lifting, I'd encourage you to incorporate the back bridge. Your lower back and hip health will pay dividends.

Progression:
Short Bridge 3x50
Straight Bridge 3x40
Angled Bridge 3x30

Head Bridge 2x25
Half Bridge 2x20
Full Bridge 2x15
Wall Walking Down 2x10
Wall Walking Up 2x8
Closing Bridge 2x6
Stand-to-Stand Bridge 2x20

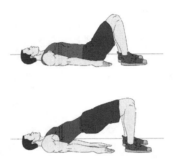

Beginner: Straight Bridge

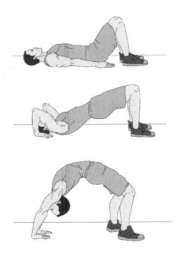

Intermediate: Full Bridge

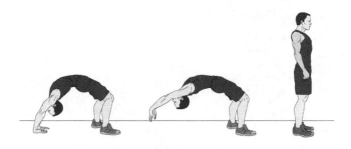

Advanced: Stand-to-Stand Bridge

Muscle Building Cardio

Early Morning Roadwork and Sprinting

If you are trying to shed body fat in the best manner possible, sprinting is an excellent way to develop your lower body power while getting you to your goal. This is not a complicated concept. Go sprint, recover, repeat. Don't die. As with your strength training, you can either train LONG or you can train HARD. You cannot do both.

A twenty to thirty-minute brisk walk first thing in the morning regardless of your fitness endeavors is a fantastic way to begin your day. This is especially true if you lack the motivation for high-intensity sprints. You could consider this Steady State cardio, but I'd prefer to call it just getting your day started right. Walking is a great lifestyle habit and it will burn a few extra calories as well as aid in recovery. You should primarily be using your diet to drive fat loss, not cardio. Getting an easy win first thing in the morning by burning a few extra calories and getting your head space right during the walk will have profound impacts on your physique as well as mind-set for the day.

Guerrilla Warfare

Being an Army guy, I can't overlook the value of jogging first thing in the morning. Though it is not essential for progress, I run because I enjoy it. Boxers and elite military units have been doing this for decades. A long jog, however, really isn't necessary or the most efficient way to get ripped.

If you're looking for an extra calorie burn after your strength training or on your "off" days, High Intensity Interval Training (HIIT) is the way to go, not a slow-burn death race. Look no further than the burpee in its various forms to leave you gasping for air, dripping with sweat, and getting you the most bang for your buck. Incinerate fat in the comfort of your hotel room, all without having to endure the elements. No excuses necessary.

Burpees: The burpee is the ultimate full-body cardio exercise. I will give you my favorite burpee workout, but if you don't feel like you need the variation, the basic burpee has been giving football teams, elite military forces, and CrossFit nerds results for a long time. To perform a basic burpee, begin in a squat position with hands on the floor in front of you. Kick your feet back to a push-up position, immediately return your feet to the squat position, leap up as high as possible from the squat position, and for good measure clap at the height of the movement. Yay burpees!

Perform the following for 12-15 reps each with as little time between exercises as possible:

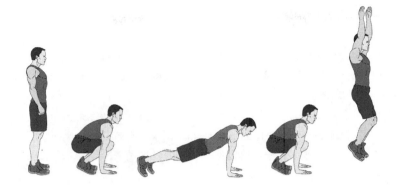

Burpee Illustrations

Standard burpee

Burpee-jax

Squat-Burpee

Chest-ground

Single-leg Mountain Climber

Side Kick-through

Chop & Hop

Angry Mule

Triple Skyfall

One-arm Getup

Yay Burpees!

Tabata Plyometrics

The ultimate fat-burning protocol that is also great for developing explosive power, improving agility, and foot speed are plyometrics programed into Tabata intervals! You can setup the Tabata protocol (20 second max effort, 10 second rest) for pretty much any exercise, but I find pairing it with a multi-joint plyometric exercise yields the best results. Find a step or sturdy bench. Jump up onto it. Jump off. Repeat this as many times as possible in 20 seconds. Rest 10 seconds and repeat 8 more times. Four minutes in hell that will make you more athletic as well as strip off fat! Simple. You thought you needed a $1,500 treadmill or stationary bike in the gym across town? Give this a try, and you won't be climbing onto another worthless elliptical again.

For fat loss you can use Tabatas or sprinting up to three times per week, but I've used up to three different Tabata intervals in one workout when pressed for time. Perform them after strength training so that you have the energy to perform your max effort on the keystone exercises mentioned above.

Most sports require you to call upon every ounce of strength you have and explode throughout the entire competition, even if you're tired. Including Tabata protocols into your workout will add to your arsenal, incinerate fat, and smoke your competition.

Nutrition Section

The thermogenic effect of food is directly proportional to the amount of calories consumed, not the frequency of feeding. It is as simple as calories in versus calories out. Really. Meal timing and frequency is actually largely irrelevant to body composition. Eating more frequently will not speed up your metabolism and burn more fat. Eating six to eight small meals per day will NOT allow you to lose fat any faster than eating two (or however many), provided the calorie/macronutrient breakdown of these meals are the same. Simplicity wins.

There are obviously more optimal and less optimal approaches to the topic of nutrition, particularly when considering training intensity, recovery, and carbohydrate partitioning. However, the most important rule regarding meal timing and body composition is to meet your individual daily macronutrient targets. Do not sacrifice carbohydrate and fat intake for the sake of eating additional protein.

I have followed the eight-meal-a-day approach, but I've made the leanest gains by eating on a schedule of two meals a day following a sixteen-hour fasting period. Be a lifestyle bodybuilder. Fitness should contribute to your life and be sustainable. Anything that doesn't add to the quality of your life detracts from it. Hit your macros and plan your day around the foods you love to eat, at a frequency that fits in with your lifestyle. You will not jeopardize your gains because you have to wait a few hours before you get to eat lunch. Eat and train intelligently. Additionally, you can fit your favorite foods into your diet if you plan ahead accordingly.

To simplify things as much as possible, some quick "rules" are as follows:

-If you're trying to loose fat, multiply your weight times 12 for total daily calories. For example, a 190-pound man would eat 2,280 calories. Enough to put him in a deficit to loose fat, but not so much that he'd be at a massive risk to lose muscle. A deficit of 3,500 calories over the WEEK is require to lose one pound.

-Conversely, if you're trying to build lean muscle, multiple your body weight time 16. For example, a 165-pound man would consume 2,640 calories. Enough to spur muscular gain with as little added fat as possible.

-Avoid processed foods, food alternatives, additives, and foods that come in a box or bag. Opt for foods that are as close to how you'd find them in nature as possible and shop for fresh, local, food every few days.

-Drink plenty of water. You don't need to be a bodybuilder-bro and carry around your gallon of water, but make sure you're consuming at least half your body weight in ounces per day.

-Limit consumption of inflammatory foods like wheat, corn, soy, and sugar. They won't kill you, but the Paleo Guys are onto something when observing a "caveman-like" diet. Don't consume foods with more than five ingredients.

-Cook with coconut or macadamia nut oil. They are tasty and loaded with healthy fats.

-Consume more carbohydrates on days that you train hard, and limit your fruit intake to 1-2 servings on days that you don't.

-Eat more vegetables in general, and consider supplementing with a Greens drink when you don't.

Apps like MyFitnessPal have revolutionized the lifestyle diet and allow us to go out to eat with loved ones while continuing to progress on our diet. I don't even consider myself on a diet. Tracking my macronutrients to support my training goals allows me to eat whatever I want, guilt free. Once you know your target numbers, it's easy to stick to your plan.

Stop using a diet designed for a pro-bodybuilder or a middle-aged housewife. Are you taking 350mg/week of testosterone with a myriad of other androgens? Or are you a middle-class housewife with three kids in your forties who thinks working out means going for a walk around the block with your girl friends? Then why are you dieting like a kale-detox sipping mommy or your favorite fitness model?

Layperson diets are designed to meet their goal — smaller numbers on the scale. Unless you're morbidly obese and trying to avoid amputation from diabetic complications, your goals probably exceed the capacity of "popular" diets' abilities. You want to be leaner, but you also want more muscle and more athletic ability. None of these can be delivered by the mass media or frozen dinner nutrition plans your parents use.

Don't take "You gotta eat big to get big" too far. There's a difference between eating enough to fuel workouts, recovery, and hypertrophy, and eating too much. Consuming a few hundred calories over maintenance is all you really need to fuel muscle gains. Take the diet advice of the USDA and pro bodybuilders with a grain of salt. You might be able to pick up a few tips from fitness gurus in magazines — many are actually pretty smart — but remember that their plans are just that: THEIR plans, not yours.

You cannot train your way out of a poor diet. Since being lean is a prerequisite to getting ripped abs, you will have to show some restraint at times. As a general rule we could all probably stand to eat more veggies and less everything else. Get rid of the obvious junk foods that are problematic for everyone. Food quality matters, but you don't need to break the bank at Whole Foods. Cooking your own food is a very basic form of self-reliance. If you can't feed yourself, then you're putting your physique goals into the hands of others — and those people don't have your best interest at heart. Even if you train regularly, you're probably limited on time and have other responsibilities, but don't let your excuses dictate your waistline. Diet must be adjusted for your specific needs and current activity level.

Eat less sugar and avoid processed, synthetic foods. "Low-fat" foods do not mean low-fat you. Be dubious of any food that makes a blatant health claim like "low-fat," "low-sugar," "gluten free" or "all natural." When a phrase like "sugar free" is the best a food conglomerate's legal team can do to convince you that their products will not kill you, then perhaps it's best to avoid the product in the first place. Stay away from anything with a long list of ingredients that you could not identify in nature, like soy lecithin or anything with the word "syrup."

Skip the juice, and just eat the fruit. Drink lots of water. The importance of drinking water cannot be overstated. Among other things, water removes the byproducts of fat and improves metabolic rate and digestion. It removes toxins and reduces aches and pains, helping you to train harder and more consistently. This helps you get leaner. Obviously, avoid soda, sugary beverages and sports drinks.

Even with the above recommendations, free yourself from the illusion that you can't eat certain foods, do certain things, or enjoy social occasions to the fullest while achieving your desired body composition. Give yourself the freedom to incorporate some of the foods and activities you love, within moderation, but try to hit your macronutrient requirements MOST of the time. Don't get frustrated by ridiculous fad diet rules that have been unnecessarily placed upon you. Give yourself the freedom to stick to your dietary plan for the long term.

Where You Are Now: Identifying Body Fat Percentage and Tracking Progress

The first step in getting where you want to go is to accurately identify where you are. This is true for land navigation as well as body composition. You need to know where you are, so you know where you're going. We are will treat the plan as a cross between a roadmap and a math equation.

The scale is a useful tool, but it is not the only way we will determine our starting point or assess progress. Taking measurements is key because changes in water, salt, and carb intake will cause variations on the scale and the tape. Weigh yourself every morning then at the end of the week calculate your average. It's best to look at the data over three to four weeks.

Finally, it is important to take progress photos the first day and every four weeks. Take two photos: one front and one side. Consistency is key to accurate tracking. This means that measurements and photos need to be taken at the same time of the day, under the same circumstances. The best time to measure is in the morning after using the toilet. Use the same lighting conditions, camera angle, and time of day. Be warned that taking progress pictures more often can be stressful as the changes are often too small to be motivational.

A quick note on the myth of spot reduction, when around 15% body fat or lower, fat comes off the upper abs first. Before that there doesn't seem to be any pattern.

The 10 Points of Measurement:

Feel free to tense/flex your muscles for each measurement as this enables more consistent results and helps you take the measurements in the same place each time. Take and note measurements to the nearest 1/16" Not only is it exceptionally useful for noting small changes and trends in the data, but without the data, you are blind after all. What can be measured can be changed.

1. Neck
2. Right bicep
3. Left bicep
4. Nipple line at chest
5. Two fingers above navel
6. Navel
7. Two fingers below navel
8. Widest point of hips
9. Widest part of right leg
10. Widest part of left leg

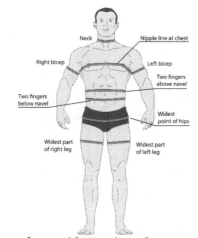

Image of man with 10 points of measurement

It is also important to track your current level of strength because strength increases correlate well to muscle gains. Muscle growth can hide fat loss, so you can't only rely on the scale to track progress. Do you weigh the same as you did last month but your strength stats are up and your stomach measurements down? If so then that's progress. It's a numbers game that we can win even if it were a zero sum game.

Macronutrients

Protein, fat, carbohydrates, and fiber!

Protein helps us to recover from our training, it preserves lean tissue, and it helps us grow more muscle; however, it is not as simple as saying more is better. The most important factor in determining our protein intake requirement is lean body mass. The leaner mass you have, the more protein you need. Basically a fatter individual can get away with less protein than a lean and muscular athlete. We can determine lean mass by taking our weight and subtracting the amount of body fat.

"Optimal" intake for physique goals is only ~.8 − 1.2 grams per pound, depending on lean body mass (LBM).

Protein intake past that range isn't likely to benefit our muscles because protein synthesis will already be maxed out. So beware of the fitness industry nonsense that would love to sell you another tub of protein powder. Just to be clear: High protein diets do not cause kidney damage and consuming too much protein will not likely be detrimental to anything other than to our wallets.

Protein powders are a useful tool to make hitting protein targets affordable, not to mention convenient. However, getting your protein intake from real food is always going to be superior. Consuming protein primarily through meat, fish, and eggs will deliver the highest quality nutrients and combat hunger.

To make things simple when just getting started, eat one gram of protein per pound or about 33% of your caloric intake from protein. Protein has four calories in every gram. With protein intake set, it's time to determine where the rest of your daily caloric intake will come from.

There are nine Calories in every gram of fat and consumption of dietary fat is important for regular hormonal function, especially testosterone production. It should never be eliminated from a diet.

You should aim to consume ~0.4 − 0.6 g/lb or 20-30% of your calories from fat.

Those carrying more body fat will do better with a higher fat in-

73

take than leaner individuals, so if you have a higher body fat percentage, go with the upper end of the range. There is room for personal preference, though. Some people simply do better with different fat intakes (which is probably also largely linked to insulin sensitivity), so feel free to experiment.

Now it's time to find out how many "fun" calories you can consume from carbohydrates. (The rest of your daily calorie intake.) There are four calories in every gram of carbohydrates. Carbs help fuel us through life and workouts, replace muscle glycogen, and make your diet a lot tastier. Even though we must limit their consumption, do not eliminate them from your diet. We need to eat enough carbohydrates to still get effective workouts so that we can maintain our muscle mass.

Fiber is a carbohydrate and eating it is important because it keeps us feeling fuller without adding significantly to the calorie content of food. It lowers blood sugar levels, delays the digestion of food, lowers cholesterol, and helps us avoid constipation. It is clearly beneficial to include fiber in your diet, and you should aim to consume a minimum of 25g/day.

In summary, a 190-pound guy at ~20% body fat would have 152 pounds of LBM (190 x .20 = 38lbs of fat)

Baseline protein intake: 152 x ~1.1 = 168g protein/day (672 calories)

Baseline fat intake: 152 x .5 = 76g fat/day (684 calories)

Carbohydrate intake = the rest of your daily calories…

It has been my experience that a healthy deficit is 12 times your body weight. Therefore 190 x 12 = 2,280 - [Calories from protein + fat (1,356)] = 924 calories from carbohydrates = 231g/day

This is your starting point. Consume these ratios of macronutrients and record your scale weight, your measurements, and your strength. Stick to the numbers for one month before you start messing with different macronutrient ratios. You need to see where you are in order to see where you're going. Use a calorie counting application like MyFitnessPal to make life a lot easier.

As mentioned earlier, if you're a skinny guy trying to pack on some lean mass, you can follow the same setup for protein and fat, however you'd take your body weight and multiply it by 16. Consume the difference in carbohydrates.

Example — a skinny 165-pound guy trying to add some size would consume 2,640 calories. (165x16)

Protein: 165 x 1 = 165g (660 calories, slightly less than the baseline protein intake above)

Fat: 165 x .5 = 82.5g (743 calories)

Carbohydrate: 2,640 (-660) (-742) = 1,238 / 4 = 310g

Intermittent Fasting

There are no magic formulas, pills, powders, or potions that will guarantee success. If there were, we would all know about it by now and everyone would walk around totally ripped. An eating strategy that has worked well for me is Intermittent Fasting. While this, too, is a sort of fad diet, I will point out to you objectively how it works for me. I like eating big, satiating meals. When I was eating small "meals" every two to three hours, I was never really full. Especially when I got down to single digit body fat and my calories dipped below 2,000 calories a day. I would be in a frenzy waiting for my "magical" feeding window to open again.

For a person looking to lose weight, intermittent fasting has a unique benefit of blunting appetite. Skipping breakfast allows for bigger, more satisfying meals later in the day that still fit your daily caloric/macronutrient requirements. Additionally, the lifestyle benefit of eating the foods you want in social settings is made possible when following this strategy. After about a week, the body's hunger hormone, ghrelin, gets used to the new eating pattern and adjusts accordingly so you no longer feel hungry in the mornings. Magic? No, but it feels like it. It is also easier to plan meals because with fewer meals to eat, there are fewer meals to prepare. Eating only two to three times a day, it's harder to screw up your macronutrient counting, and you have more time in your day to enjoy your life without stressing over food.

Base the time you train on when you feel the strongest and have time to do it. If you train late in the day, make sure that you have time to eat a meal afterward. On the days you train, have the majority of the calories after the workout. As a rule of thumb, try to eat within two hours after your training. However, the key is to keep things as simple as possible and just eat two to three meals per day.

Here are two strategies I've used with intermittent fasting:

Training after work
12:00 Snack (~20% calories/macros)
2:00-3:00 Strength training
3:30 Afternoon/Post-workout meal (20-40% calories/macros)
7:30 Dinner (remaining calories/macros)

Training first thing in the morning
7:00-8:00 Strength Training
11:00 Lunch (~50% calories/macros)
7:00 Dinner (~50% calories/macros)

... Or if I'm not training that day
12:00 Lunch (~40% calories/macros)
7:30 Dinner (~60% calories/macros)
Easy, peasy.

Supplements

I'm not going to sugarcoat it; most supplements are total bullshit.

I do believe in the benefits of caffeine for its hunger suppressing abilities as well as increasing intensity and focus… but you can get all these benefits from a strong cup of coffee. The only supplement I would recommend is MAYBE branched chain amino acids if you must train early in the morning or fasted. Supplements are not necessary to accomplish your goals. Eating health food that fits your macronutrient needs will.

However, if you're interested in getting highly technical and want to spend the cash on supplements that may affect 5% of your total progress, I'll lay out a schedule that I did see results from. Again, this is advanced, and absolutely not necessary if you have your diet and training dialed in. I have spent thousands of dollars and hours upon hours reading scientific journals still playing the trial and error game to come up with the following:

- Athletic Greens or similar drink if you don't get enough vegetables during the day

- Spicy metabolism boosting/liver detoxing drink on an empty stomach:

¼ cup Apple Cider Vinegar

½ squeezed lemon

¼ tbs cinnamon

¼ tbs cayenne peper

½ tbs organic honey

20oz ice water

If you train fasted, take 10g BCAAs roughly 10minutes pre-workout, then 10g BCAAs every two hours until you eat your first meal of the day.

Other than that, try to get your protein and vitamins from whole food sources and stay away from all the marketing ploys to feed you over processed and overhyped snake oil.

All in all, it's calories in versus calories out — train hard and get stronger.

I do not endorse any specific supplement company, and I opt to make my own by buying them in bulk if I take any at all. There are a few worthwhile supplements out there, and I recommend you look for ones that contain the following.

PRE-WORKOUT:

Phase 1 – Taken 45 Minutes Prior To Training:
- BCAA Powder: 5 g
- Glycine: 1 g
- L-Citrulline/DL-Malate 4g
- DMG 500mg
- Maltodextrin: 20 g
- MCT Oil: 1 Tbsp
- Creatine Monohydrate: 5 g
- Sugar-Free Powdered Drink Mix (like Kool-Aid)
- 12 oz. water

Phase 2 – Taken 15 Minutes Prior To Training:
- 12 oz. water
- Caffeine: 100mg
- Strong Black Coffee – One 8-oz. cup

(Note: If you don't like coffee, simply chew up one 200 mg caffeine tablet instead of the 100mg + coffee)

INTRA-WORKOUT:
- BCAA Powder: 10 g
- Maltodextrin: 20 g
- Caffeine Anhydrous: 200 mg
- N-Acetyl L-Tyrosine 400mg
- L-Carnosine: 500 mg
- L-Glutamine: 5 g
- Potassium Bicarbonate: 1 g
- Sugar-Free Powdered Drink Mix (like Kool-Aid)
- Sugar substitute (like Splenda)
- 1 liter bottle filled with water

FAT BURNER:

Formula 1 (Once/Day):
• Green Tea Extract: 300 mg EGCG
• Caffeine Anhydrous: 200 mg
Formula 2 (3 Times/Day):
• Conjugated Linoleic Acid: 1 g x 3
• Acetyl L-Carnitine 425mg
• Alpha Lipoic Acid 200mg
• Fish Oil/Omega 3
• (Containing 180mg EPA/120mg DHA): 1 g x 3
• Organic Flax Oil: 1 tsp x 3

PM HORMONE BOOSTER: 45 minutes before bed
• Arginine Alpha Ketoglutarate: 5g
• L-Lysine 680mg
• DL-Methionine 1g
• Gamma Aminobutyric Acid: 5 g
• Zinc: 15 mg
• Melatonin: 3g
• BCAA Powder: 10 g

**Take 2-5 grams of creatine with somewhere between 100-250 mg cinnamon extract powder right before and immediately after your workouts.

**Take 3-5 grams L-arginine or arginine alpha-ketoglutarate twice a day, away from other

protein meals, with 3 grams of HMB. If possible, time one of your doses 30–60 minutes

before your workout and the other 30-60 minutes before bed.

**Take 60-100 grams of simple carbohydrates right after your workout, along with 1-1.5 grams of fenugreek.

**Take 5-10 grams of glutamine 2–4 times per day on an empty stomach. Take two of the four doses before and after your workout along with .5 grams of carnosine.

**Take 20 grams of whey protein immediately before training and 20-40 grams immediately after — along with 5 grams of leucine, either by itself or from branched-chain amino acids (BCAAs). If you go with BCAAs, make sure that the product has at least 5 grams of leucine, 2.5 grams of isoleucine, and 2.5-5 grams of valine per dose.

You can purchase all of these supplements in bulk and make your own for 25% of what the big supplement companies charge. You won't get any "proprietary blends" or additives you don't want to consume if you do it this way. However, all you really need is a couple of cups of strong coffee and a protein shake if you're in a pinch to supplement your healthy diet.

Alcohol, BPA, Soy

Calories that come from alcohol aren't really going to assist your body in any way. That being said, it isn't going to totally destroy your progress either. The human body is surprisingly resilient, and strong people have been consuming alcohol for a long, long time. Alcohol itself isn't so much a fat storer as it is a fat-burning suppressor. If your goal is fat loss, getting yourself out of that mode for several hours isn't wise. Heavy drinking has several mechanisms that will inhibit muscle-protein synthesis and recovery.

My advice is that if you're going to drink, you should try to make it fit into your macros. Just be forewarned that you are essentially taking away from calories that could be assisting you with training and recovery. Calories aside, a beer or two after work or on the weekend obviously isn't going to ruin your physique. But as such, your weight loss and strength gaining efforts will be inhibited to a certain extent. Choosing to disregard and have a big night out is likely going to mean you'll be consuming far too many calories for the day, and your workout the following day will suffer. Regardless, it's your life and progress over the long term. Think bigger picture. What's the point of achieving the body of your dreams if you can't enjoy yourself in the process of getting and maintaining it?

Alcohol is its own macronutrient that contains 7 calories per gram. However, if you wish to account for the calories you're drinking and fit a beer, etc. into your macros, simply apply the following:

Use your carb macros – divide the total calories of the drink you're consuming (total calories, not just the calories from any carbs or fats in the drink) by 4 and simply use as grams of carbs.

As an example, a 144-calorie beer would be calculated as 36g of carbs. (144 divided by 4)

My strategy is just to consume no more than three drinks in one sitting. Alcohol has been shown to interfere with sleep quality, so if you're going to drink, try to cut it off three hours before going to bed. Another strategy I use is to make sure I have eaten dinner before I drink. A full belly will prevent you from overdoing it on the booze. Consuming supplements or alcohol on an empty stomach will allow the body to metabolize it much faster which translates to reduced dosage effectiveness.

BPA, or bisphenol A, is a widely studied and scientifically agreed upon endocrine disruptor. It leaches into the human body from nearly all polycarbonate plastic products, drink containers, sporting equipment, epoxy resins, and the lining of food cans. It is literally everywhere, and is almost guaranteed to be having a negative effect on your testosterone levels.

BPA is used to line the inside of food cans. Opt for fresh or frozen foods instead. Stop eating foods that are packaged in BPA-laden cans and polycarbonate plastic food containers with the number 7 on them (recycling code). Use glass, porcelain, or stainless steel cookware to store and heat your food.

Traditional sales receipts contain high levels of BPA. When your cashier asks if you'd like your receipt, politely decline or ask them to put it your bag for you. To make matters worse, hand sanitizer has been found to speed up absorption of BPA. A study found that subjects had abnormally high serum BPA levels and BPA in their urine after handling receipts with "sanitized" hands. Stick to good old fashioned soap and water before you eat.

Soy is one of the most heavily genetically modified foods on the planet. It has been shown to reduce testosterone levels in men and increase estrogen levels in women. Soy is not worth your time or money, and it's definitely not worth your health. The risks that come with consuming soy products far outweigh any potential benefits in your "low fat" protein cereal.

Sample Meal Plan

I'm a huge fan of crock-pot cooking. Not only is it simple and delicious, it's easy to batch cook a lot of healthy food as well as clean up quickly. There is very little skill required to make a delicious and healthy meal that will feed you for multiple days.

Simple rules to a successful slow cooker meal are to follow a "Green/Face Diet." If it's green or had to die for your dietary needs, it's in!

1. Get a giant hunk of animal flesh: beef roast, a dozen chicken breasts, a turkey breast, or a couple of pork tenderloins.

2. Salt and pepper or slather meat with tomato paste.

3. Vegetables/greens. Chop them up. Throw them in. Frozen veggies work too.

4. Depending on your macros, dice up some potatoes and add them to the pot.

5. Add liquid. I suggest stock, any kind: beef, chicken, or vegetable.

In the morning, turn your cooker on low for 7-8 hours. Now go live your life and do the things you love to do: work, school, smashing heads, whatever. Come home and it'll be ready for a feast. If applicable, store the leftovers for later.

Nutrient-Dense Chili Recipe

- 3 pounds grass-fed ground beef or turkey
- 1-2 medium onions, chopped
- 2 red peppers, chopped
- 5 carrots, chopped
- 2 cups spinach
- 2 cloves garlic, minced
- 28 ounces Italian peeled tomatoes with juice
- 46 ounces Spicy Hot V8 Juice
- 16 ounces red kidney beans, drained
- 16 ounces white northern beans, drained
- 2 tsp iodized salt (to protect you from all-too-common iodine deficiencies)
- 2 tsp oregano
- 5 tsp. chili powder
- ¾ tsp red pepper flakes
- 1 cup raw cashews, ground until almost butter

Optional: one-fourth pound grass-fed liver, ground to itty-bitty bits (this small of an amount won't affect the taste)

1. Brown burger (and liver, if so desired) in large soup kettle and remove when cooked.
2. Brown onions, red peppers, carrots, and garlic in olive oil in the same kettle.
3. Add tomatoes, V8 juice, beans, all the spices, and the ground cashews and stir.
4. Cover and simmer for at least two hours, stirring occasionally.
5. Add spinach about 10 minutes before eating.

The Standard Meat & Potatoes

- Potatoes
- Ground beef
- Tomato sauce

- Sea salt (to taste)

1. Chop and cook the potatoes in a crock pot until soft.
2. When ready, cook the ground beef in a skillet, season with some sea salt, and stir in the tomato sauce.
3. Smash some soft potatoes into a big bachelor sized bowl and add the sloppy beef with tomato sauce on top and enjoy.

Sweet Potato Hash

- Sweet potatoes
- Onions
- Green peppers
- Rotisserie chicken
- Curry seasoning (optional)

1. Dice the sweet potatoes into cubes, boil in water until soft.
2. In another skillet, sauté the peppers and onions in olive oil or butter.
3. When ready, pile the soft diced sweet potatoes into a mountain on your plate and put the sautéed peppers and onions on top.
4. Now pile a bunch of chicken (with the skin) on top of that and season with whatever spice you want.

Steak and Eggs

- Steak
- Eggs

Instructions: Cook steak. Cook eggs. Put on same plate. Eat.

Crispy Shepherd's Pie

- Russet potatoes

- Olive oil (or coconut oil)
- Sea Salt
- Ground beef
- Cheese

1. Slice the potatoes in wedges and sprinkle with oil.
2. Bake on oven sheet until crispy brown. Take out and apply sea salt.
3. Cook ground beef in a skillet until ready.
4. Layer the crispy potatoes on a plate, then put the ground beef on top.
5. Melt some slices of cheese over your pile of food. Enjoy.

Hawaiian Pulled Pork

- Pork shoulder
- Pineapple
- BBQ Sauce

1. Cook the pork in a slow cooker until it is tender.
2. Dice the pineapples and stir together with BBQ sauce.
3. Smother the pork in the Pineapple/BBQ sauce.

Crockpot Beef Stew

- Beef tips
- Beef stock
- Carrots
- Onions
- Peppers

1. Chop veggies
2. Add stock and beef tips all into crock pot.
3. Cook until ready.

Steak Fajitas

- Skirt steak strips
- Onions
- Peppers
- Avocado
- Cheese
- Potatoes

1. Slice potatoes into wedges and sprinkle with melted coconut oil and salt.
2. Bake until crispy brown.
3. Sauté steak, onions, peppers in a skillet.
4. Slice fresh avocado and grate cheese.
5. Eat steak and veggies with crispy potatoes on the side.
6. Put avocado slices and cheese on top. Add salsa.

The Bird's Nest

- Potatoes
- Greek yogurt
- Rotisserie Chicken
- Eggs

1. Bake or boil the potatoes
2. Mash them up with some Greek yogurt and salt and pepper.
3. Cook the eggs over-easy.
4. Make a pile of potatoes on the plate, put the eggs on top of the pile, then put some pieces of chicken on top. Viola, a bird's nest!

Spanish Beef

- Ground beef
- Shredded cheese

- Avocado
- Salsa
- White rice

1. In a skillet, cook the beef.
2. Serve over rice with salsa and fresh avocado.

Crock Pot Cheesy Potatoes

- Potatoes
- Cheese
- Ground beef

1. Chop potatoes and cook in water in a crock pot.
2. Cook beef in a skillet.
3. When ready, melt cheese over potatoes and serve with beef.

Lean-Body Chocolate Peanut Butter Fudge Recipe

- ¾ cup organic canned coconut milk
- 1 bar (3-5 oz. bar works well) of bakers unsweetened chocolate — 100% cacao content
- 4-5 tablespoons of organic peanut butter or your favorite nut butter
- ¾ cup raisins or dried cranberries
- ½ cup whole raw almonds or other nuts
- ⅓ cup raw chopped pecans
- 1 scoop, about 25g of your favorite protein powder
- 3 Tbsp chia seeds and/or flax seeds
- 1 teaspoon vanilla extract
- A little natural stevia powder to sweeten or a small touch of real maple syrup (1-2 Tbsp max)

1. Start by adding the coconut milk and vanilla extract to a small saucepan on VERY low heat — the lowest heat setting.
2. Break up the extra dark chocolate bar into chunks and add into pot. Add the nut butters and the stevia, and continuously stir until it all melts together into a smooth mixture.
3. Add the raisins or cranberries, nuts, seeds, protein powder, etc. and stir until fully blended.
4. If the mixture becomes too thick or has a dry consistency, just add a small amount more coconut milk. If the mixtures seems too wet, keep in mind that it will solidify a good bit once it goes in the fridge.
5. Spoon/pour the fudge mixture onto some waxed paper in a dish and place in the fridge until it cools and solidifies together (3-4 hours).
6. Cut into squares once firm and place in a closed container or cover with foil in fridge to prevent it from drying out.

Enjoy small squares of this delicious healthy "super-food" fudge for dessert and for small snacks.

No-Bake Protein Poppers

- Natural Peanut Butter: 1 ⅓ Cup
- Blackstrap Molasses: 1 Tbsp
- Vanilla Whey Protein Isolate Powder: 1 ¼ Cups
- Raw Oat Bran: 1 Cup (If you can't find Oat Bran, blend "quick cook" rolled oats in a blender until very fine)
- Ground Flax Meal: 2 Tbsp
- Powdered Cinnamon: 1 Tsp

Optional Ingredients:
Dark Chocolate Chips, Raw Nuts (Almonds, Peanuts, Walnuts, Etc.), Dried Fruit (Raisins, Cranberries, Banana Chips, etc.)

1. Mix the peanut butter and molasses in a large bowl and microwave for about 1 minute. (If making less than a full batch,

reduce microwave time accordingly; i.e., ½ batch = 30 seconds.)

2. Combine the remaining ingredients in a separate bowl and mix together thoroughly. Add the peanut butter mixture and mix with your hands (have fun!) until completely mixed. "Scrunch" the mixture in your hands, forming small balls slightly larger than the size of quarter and place them on a plate to let stand about 20 minutes. Place covered in a refrigerator and pop 4 of them into a baggie or plastic container for a take-along meal replacement treat!

Setting You Up to Win

Warming up prior to intense training is critical. Run through a few dynamic stretches if you train hard, fast, and are in it for the long term. If you don't have time to warm up, you don't have time to train. Lubricating your joins with blood will allow you to become more flexible, and it will save you from injury. Elevating your heart rate and internal temperature will allow you to get the most out of the subsequent workout. Here are a few drills you can run through in five to ten minutes before you start to train.

Loosen up the hips, hamstrings, and glutes with some Leg Swings.

Begin with forward leg swings. Find something to hold for balance if you need to. Swing your right leg backward and forward as high and as far back as you can. Do 20 swings on each leg before moving onto side-to-side swings. Swing your right leg out to the side as high as possible and then in front of you toward your left as far as you can. Again, perform 20 swings on each leg. Repeat all four moves one more time.

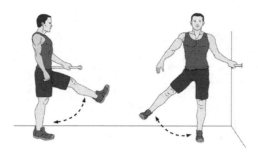

Leg swings

Next up is the Iron Cross Twist on the floor. 10 Twists.

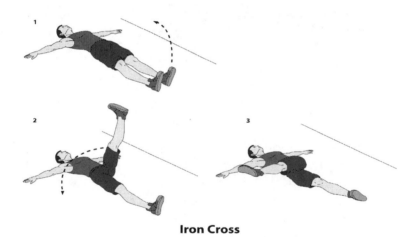

Iron Cross

Finally do some rollovers into V-sit.

This exercise is rather difficult to illustrate but simple in execution. It is like a rocking chair in motion, the spine being the rocker. The body is doubled up as shown in the illustration and this position is held as you go back. At the top of the movement, release your legs into a V and stretch briefly between your hips. Don't hold your breath, but breathe as naturally as possible. Perform 10 rollovers and then crush your workout!

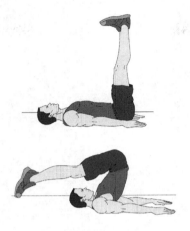

Rollover-Into V-Sit

Becoming Bendy

I've always wanted to do a split between two chairs like Jean-Claude van Damme in Blood Sport. I've not yet reached this level of flexibility, but where there is a will there is a way! Flexibility isn't something that happens overnight. I like to stretch right before bed. It's relaxing and that's generally when I'm the most limber. If you're actively trying to develop flexibility, I suggest stretching for ten to twenty minutes a day. It took me about two months of ten to twenty minutes of solid stretching every day to be able to achieve a full forward split, albeit one that was still hard to do and had to be supported with my hands.

Butterfly Position

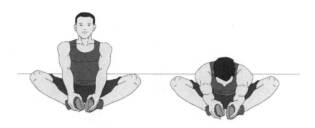

Butterfly

Keeping an arched back, lean forward like you're trying to touch your nose to your feet. While you're doing this, draw your heels ever closer to your groin. Push down on your knees with your hands and feel those hips open up.

Hips forward, legs back split progression.

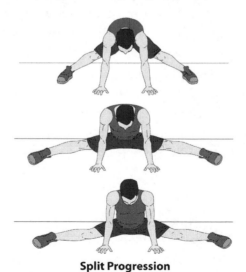

Split Progression

Side Split Progression

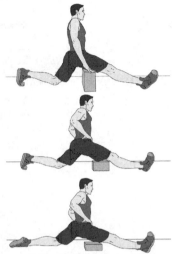

Side-Split Progression

Adjusting the stretch so that the insides of your ankles are on the floor. This makes the stretch focus on the hip joints. Resting on your heels is easier, but the stress is placed on your hamstrings. The side split will likely take longer to achieve than the forward split, but the key is to push your hips forward and be patient!

Additional valuable stretches to include in your pursuit of becoming bendy are:

Side Twists

Sit in a cross-legged position. Sit up straight and slowly turn as far around as you can.

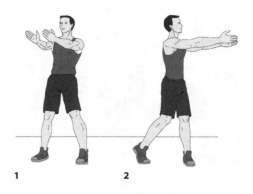

1   2

Side Twist

Side Bends

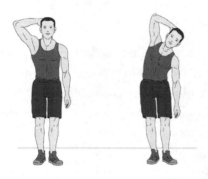

Side Bend

Toe Touches: Actually touching your toes is optional, but it's a convenient way to measure your progress.

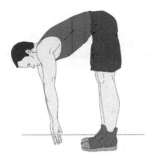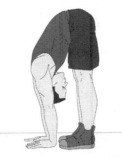

Toe-Touch Hamstring Stretch

PVC/foam rolling can also be beneficial after muscles are fully warmed up. I also enjoy performing self-myofascial release techniques with a lacrosse ball on tight knots on my back. For a more in-depth view of SMR, I'd recommend internet research of Kelly Starrett's Mobility WOD and more simply www.painscience.com/articles/tennis-ball.php

Energy and Testosterone: Going Feral

When I was going through intensive training with the United States Army, a lot of the training involved sleep deprivation. The cadre explained that the reasoning was that fatigue increases fear. The more tired we were, the more we'd have to confront our fear; these anxieties being various forms of painful death. Now that I'm living a comfortable civilian life, I don't want to experience as much daily terror. I like naps. I like a cool glass of water when I'm thirsty. When I feel stress now, I realize it isn't caused by imminent threats of violence. It is simply an adverse reaction to normal stimuli because my body is imbalanced. Maybe I'm tired because I didn't sleep enough for the rigors of everyday training and life. Maybe I'm putting my body into a frightened state and simply need to breathe more deeply. I might need to just check my posture or get up and move.

The fact is, your sleep quality is like your diet. Whether you realize it or not, it's either working for you or against you. Not sleeping enough or sleeping poorly for too long has been shown to have unavoidable and dire consequences. Conversely, good sleep habits are like a good exercise routine, and the benefits can be truly epic. Your memory improves, and you learn as well as solve problems better. With good sleep, you can stick to diets easier, your mood is generally better, and your athletic performance improves. Finally, you're also likely to live longer because your immune system functions better as well as having overall lower levels of systemic inflammation.

Create a Morning Routine

My favorite benefit of sleep is element number one in energy and testosterone production. Your goal is to have slept for seven to nine hours and ideally wake up before your alarm with a raging erection. If this is not the case, you have to re-arrange your priorities in life. If you want to sleep better, don't look to sleep aids like Melatonin. Simply commit on going to bed at a certain hour, take responsibility, and show up on time like you would for anything else that is important in your life.

I'd encourage you to start your day with a powerful morning routine that will have you moving in the direction toward success and optimal testosterone production as well as cortisol reduction. A good morning routine actually starts the night before. What gets scheduled gets done. Make sleep a priority.

Element number two is to get out of bed and start moving. I mentioned in an early chapter that I like going for a twenty to thirty-minute walk first thing in the morning. I make it a habit to roll out of my bed, right into my sweat pants and tennis shoes. It's automatic and too easy to get in this habit. It's a classic lifestyle habit I'd encourage you to include in your practice to achieve an awesome physique.

Third, is a habit of many top-performing individuals: Meditation. Start with five minutes and work your way up to fifteen to twenty minutes. Yes, you will have to get up earlier for all of these activities. I never said any of this would be easy, but it is simple!

Fourth is what I like to call The Energizer. Sit down comfortably. You should already be in position from your meditation. Relax and breathe from the abdominal region — not too shallow, not too deep. Think of it like breathing into your balls. Do this thirty times. The goal is to let the oxygen saturate not only the lungs but all of your processes. When you feel the saturation throughout your body, exhale completely and hold your breath with empty lungs. When you finally must, inhale fully and hold it for ten seconds. Repeat this two more times. You will find that by practicing this you will be able to hold each breath longer and get deeper into your body's systems. Record your results, and you'll be amazed at how long you can train yourself to hold your breath.

Increased blood oxygen circulation aids metabolism and creates more energy throughout all your systems. To complete The Energizer, take two or three deep breaths, entirely emptying lungs, and then filling them to their fullest capacity. Stand up, reach upward keeping elbows and knees straight, fists clinched. Stretch upward with your feet comfortably apart the width of your shoulders. Bring the body from position A to position B repeatedly in a controlled manner. Lift chin up while standing but avoid leaning backward. Inhale slowly through the nose until the lungs are completely filled, elevate the shoulders as high as you can and draw the abdominal walls inward to a stomach vacuum. Then release abdominal walls and bring the body into position B exhaling through the nose, bending the knees, and bringing the armpits close to the knees attempting to touch the floor with the hands about eighteen inches from the feet. Repeat fifteen times.

You may be seeing stars at this point. This is your body's energy being released. Use it to live an inspired life. Get after it.

Also, don't forget to hydrate to eliminate the impurities you just released from within. You don't need to drink a gallon of water a day like the gym bros, but staying fully hydrated has innumerable benefits. You should be urinating once per hour through the working day.

Speaking of water, just for good measure, I would encourage you to build some mental toughness and purposeful suffering with a cold shower before you head into work. Take a cold shower to finish your morning routine, and start your day with some intensity! Raising your core temperature will amplify the tonic effect of a cold shower upon the nervous system. So to gain the maximum benefit of these cold showers, you should aim to precede them with sufficient exercise.

Beginner Bodyweight Routine:

A Newfound Respect for Gravity

A quick note about programming — limiting my intense training to an every-other-day schedule has been the key to my strength gaining protocol. This is ideal for people who have lives outside of the gym and allows for a balanced training to rest ratio. I recommend three to four days a week of training to everyone, no matter their level of fitness.

"The only difference between a rut and a grave is the depth." - Unknown

Once upon a time, I was training in the gym six to seven days a week. I would struggle to gain strength and would plateau often. I believed I just needed to keep swinging the hammer, and if the nails weren't going in, I just had to swing the hammer harder. It takes roughly forty-eight hours of rest from heavy training to allow your nervous system to recharge fully. My muscles may not have felt sore, but my central nervous system was never given the rest it needed in order to recover. Strength training doesn't only tax the specific muscles you are using, and if you're not recovering from your workouts, you're effectively taking three steps backward for every two forward.

If you take nothing else from this book, consider reducing training frequency, getting very strong at four to six exercises, and finishing off your muscles with some bodyweight finishers. I'm laying out an all bodyweight plan, but pursuing a one-arm chin-up is a noble pursuit even in a standard weight training regimen. Once you are able to pull yourself over the bar under control with one arm, your biceps will swell and your back will be forced to widen. If you train properly, developing substantial muscle is totally achievable with or without weights.

Cancel Your Gym Membership!

Cancel your gym membership and stop the constant wheel spinning of your current weight lifting regimen. I know weights are kind of sexy, and the cable pulldown machine is shiny. I know the bench press and power rack look really cool. If you are willing to put in the effort, you can build strength and muscle without any external weights at all. I prefer calisthenics to weights for many reasons. I am not anti-weightlifting. It is by far a much healthier form of exercise than pure cardio like running, especially if you're trying to build a powerful physique.

There is no one way to achieve fitness, and I just want to share with you a different approach to achieve your genetic potential without spending hours picking things up and putting them down until inevitable injury occurs. It's also really easy to go to the gym and work out every day of the week using weights performing isolation lifts. This stress on your system over long periods of time leads to a chronic level of cortisol in your system. I love to exercise every day, and I am not saying you shouldn't. It definitely feels great to exercise, but research shows constant lifting day in day out is not ideal.

Fitness is free and to be honest, gym memberships are expensive. Seriously, $30 - $200+ a month supporting your gym habit? Depending on where you live, this could go to use in much more beneficial ways in your life. What do you do when you travel? Do you change your goals or do you skip working out entirely? If you decide you're going to pursue bodyweight mastery, you're in luck. You can make progress anywhere in the world!

Unless you are meticulous about your form and movement, weight lifting often leads to injury and disproportionate looks. The big traditional barbell powerlifting may transfer well to football, but when was the last time you were running up and down the grid-iron? These lifts do generally keep your whole body working together, but injuries still occur far more often than anyone would like to admit.

Additionally, people run into problems when they start isolating body parts and taking the training programs from popular articles in magazines and Internet forums. "Should I lift 3x10 at 75% 1RM? Or 5x5 at 85% 1RM?" There are countless other sets and rep variations that fitness gurus claim to be the "best" way to exercise. But I have found the quickest, most effective way to develop full-body explosive power and an aesthetically pleasing physique is to ditch the weight rack and head to the playground.

It's free, but I think the main reason people don't train there is because it is difficult! It is not fun to face the reality of how weak you really are. You might be able to curl sixty-pound dumbbells, but what does that do for you besides being good at curling dumbbells?

It requires a little creativity and dedication, but playground workouts work your muscles very deeply. It is perplexing to me how people are content to put in endless sets and reps at their local gym with minimal results, especially when manipulating your own body actually ends up giving you the most appealing aesthetic of rock hard, dense muscle. Don't wish it was easier, wish you were better!

The beauty of bodyweight workouts is that it's almost impossible to over train. Since a full-body workout will challenge your muscles to work together deeply, the self-limiting nature of this type of training is perfect. I highly recommend just listening to your body. If you feel recovered after a day, then go back and do another full body workout. If it takes a few days to recover, then wait as long as you need in order to go back and make progress.

It isn't about how often you TRAIN it's about how often you can PROGRESS! Just do some walking, stretching, or sprinting to stay active while you recover. While the best workout regimen is no regimen at all, I've also made progress following a "Push-Pull" routine when I started getting pretty advanced in my training. Following an Upper-Lower routine allowed me to make progress when full body became too much. Advanced bodybuilders use this setup, the world around, to become brutally strong. If you're new to bodyweight training, however, you'll be better served to train more frequently with a full-body routine.

I encourage you to start with a full-body regimen because ultimately strength is a skill. The more often you practice your strength skills, the faster progress you'll make. Instead of a "chest" day once a week = 52 practices a year, a full body workout three times a week would have you training your chest strength skills 156 times! That's three times more opportunity for growth and development of the neuro pathways to get truly strong.

I like training in the following fashion:

1 "Push" exercise, 1 "Pull" exercise, 1 "Leg" exercise, and 1 "Core" exercise

It looks something like this:

Workout 1:
Push-up Progression
Pull-up Progression
Pistol Progression
L-Sit Progression

Optional - Standing Calf Raise off Step & Grip Work

Day Off
Active Rest: Walking, sprinting, stretching, and meditation

Workout 2:
Handstand Push-up Progression
Row Progression
Bridge Progression
Hanging Leg Raise Progression

Optional - Neck/Wrestler's Bridge Progressions & Calf Work

Day Off
Active Rest: Get a life!

However, if your progress levels plateau or you're experiencing an exceptionally stressful period in your life, avoid over-stressing your body parts by following a push-pull routine. I don't think overtraining is all that common and it requires pushing yourself to physical extremes, which doesn't happen too often. However, it's easy to over-stress body parts in a short amount of time and thus hamper recovery/progress.

Push-pull avoids limiting progress by grouping all the muscles involved in pulling (back, biceps, rear delts, traps, forearms, hamstrings) and all the muscles involved in pushing (chest, triceps, quads, lateral and medial delts) together. While I would encourage you to stick to full-body routines as long as you can because they increase overall physical fitness and burn more fat by training more muscles, separating your body parts by function, you're able to continue to progress when you'd otherwise become stuck or frustrated. You might short-change certain muscle groups training in this fashion, so ensure you vary the order in which the movements are performed and prioritize making progress in all your big movements.

If you're a beginner or new to bodyweight exercises, you should focus on just mastering the progressions and doing two to three work sets for each movement. Shoot for short rest periods – sixty to ninety seconds in between sets. In contrast, advanced trainers might want to add some extra volume at the end of their very strongest planned workout days by doing drop sets to easier progressions or even including a rest-paused set at the end of the movement.

I love including rest pause to my sets which look similar to this:

Decline Diamond Push-up to failure = 9 reps. Stop, take five deep breaths, and try again = 3 reps. Stop, take five more deep breaths, and repeat until failure again = 2 reps. I would total this in my journal as "RP14" and the next time I worked that movement, I would have to beat my number.

If you were to train with weights, you'd want to pick a weight that brought you to failure after your three rest-paused sets in the eleven to fifteen range. When training with body weight, we have to go for a little higher rep range since we can't simply add five pounds to the bar every week... we are moving our entire bodies through space.

Pick exercise progressions that allow you to fail in the rest-paused method in the twenty to twenty-five rep range before you advance to a more challenging progressive leverage. This allows for your tendons, joints, and ligaments to catch up with your rapidly growing muscles.

When you've gotten all you can out of a full-body split, here is how I set up my push-pull workouts.

Push-Pull Split:

Push:
Chest – Push-up Progressions
Shoulders – Handstand Progressions
Triceps – Dips/Muscle Up Progression
Quadriceps – Pistol Progressions
Calves – Standing Calf Raise on step

Day Off
Active rest: Walking, stretching, meditating

Pull:
Back Width – One Handed Pull-up Progressions
Back Thickness – Row Progressions
Biceps/Forearms – Negative Chins/Grip Progressions
Hamstrings/Glutes/Low Back – Bridge Progressions
Neck – Wrestler Bridge Progressions

Day Off
Active Rest

I consistently come back to the full-body workout time and time again. Whether I'm training with weights or only my body weight, I make the most progress when I train my body as a unit. I program my training around two workouts that mirror my favorite weight-training split:

Workout A:
Bench Press
Squat
Pull-up
Lateral Raise
Dumbbell Curl

Workout B:
Push Press
Deadlift
Row
Dip
Barbell Curl

Build A Bodacious Butt!!

The following plan will get your glutes much sexier, stronger, and functional. A vertical jump involves maximal vertical propulsion of the butt, and sprinting activates 234% more mean gluteus maximus muscle than a vertical jump. Squats and deadlifts aren't the best exercises for building bigger, stronger glutes, and most people can contract their glutes harder during bodyweight exercises than during their max weighted squats, deads, or lunges. Your glutes are typically dormant and underused, but have tons of potential power. The gluteus maximus muscles are the most important muscles in sport, and guys and girls can appreciate a well-developed hiney.

Perform these two exercises and perform two sets of ten reps with a five-second isometric hold up top after your normal leg strengthening exercise:

Bird Dog

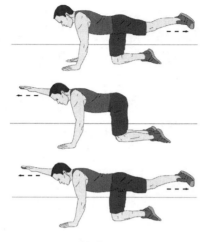

Bird Dog

Single-Leg Glute Bridge

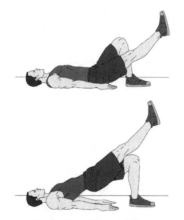

Single Leg Glute Bridge

Unlock the Power of Your Hiey's Strength through Speed

Increase your locomotive capacity with repeated of 100-meter sprints. As mentioned before, you can perform them on your "off" days or after your normal training: three to five sprints, three to five times a week.

You'll notice increased butt recruitment while running. You should maintain good sprinter form and feel them burning in your glutes and not your quads. Spend about twenty minutes warming up and progressively increase speed as the sets progress. Use a stopwatch and see if you can set a personal record.

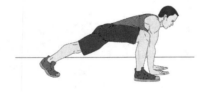

Sprinter Posture (focus on glutes/butt)

In Conclusion

Athletes have used bodyweight training techniques for centuries before barbells, machines, or steroids were ever thought of. The Greek and Roman statues of Adonis had to be modeled for and they didn't develop those bodies with high-rep crunches or jumping jacks. They pushed their bodies' limits with brutal calisthenics. You can develop your body into peak shape in the same way. Moving your body weight through space against gravity will increase strength, increase muscle mass, improve coordination for sports, injury proof tendons and ligaments, and connect your mind to your muscles through willpower and creativity. In other words, this kind of training is difficult to master, but it is the ultimate pursuit for anyone who is committed to the challenge.

Most of the exercises I recommend you master would send typical bodybuilders running for the hills. The majority of weighted movements used in typical bodybuilding routines are fairly low skill. For example, compare a seated machine press to a free-standing handstand push-up. Who is really stronger?

How long can you reasonably justify a 5,000-calorie diet as a body-builder? How are you going to stay motivated when you injure yourself with a 500-pound squat? Push-ups, pull-ups, and pistol squats will seem easier than ever when you get back to sustainable food intake. Walking up the steps will be easier when you get lighter.

If you take away nothing else from this book, I encourage you to focus on strength first with compound movements of at least two muscles from now on. Intensity and setting personal records consistently wins over meaningless repetitions. Performing the repetitions perfectly is more important than advancing to the next level in the progression.

> *"Repetition is the mother of learning, the father of action, which makes it the architect of accomplishment."*
> *~Zig Ziglar*

Fuel your body right. Your goals should be realistic and sustainable, which works out to one to two pounds a week whether you're bulking or cutting. Don't compare yourself to others. Be patient and do not constantly switch your routine around. Keep your program simple, Stupid, and keep a training log so you can see your progress over time.

> *"It doesn't matter how slowly you go so long as you do not stop." ~Confucius*

Be present in the moment and remind yourself of all the reasons "why" you're doing these exercises. Turn off your cell phone, know what you're trying to accomplish, and improve your mental attitude and focus. Having the right motivations and people around you will help with willpower. Do your best to remove temptations and distractions from your goals. Manage your stress with walking, meditating, and deep breathing.

"If you love life, don't waste time, for time is what life is made up of" ~Bruce Lee

The most advanced training machine in the world is the human body. You can develop the V-taper women love, gain a three-dimensional back, and maximize the power of your central nervous system all with bodyweight exercises. Remember that leg exercises are just as important as your "beach muscles," and that keeping a tight ass will allow you to get one or two more reps in on each exercise.

"If you are not willing to risk the unusual, you will have to settle for the ordinary." ~Jim Rohn

Maybe just try something new. I mean, variety is the spice of life! Instead of jumping on the next CrossFit bandwagon, take a step back to master the basics that you have at your disposal all times — your body versus the pull of Earth's gravity.

If nothing else, I'd challenge you to include some bodyweight alternatives to your favorite gym-rat exercises for a few weeks to appreciate the power of calisthenics.

Try — Walking Push-up instead of Bench Press.

A lot of bodybuilders like to adjust the bench press to different angles over several sets and "hit all the muscle fibers of the pectorals and front deltoids." You don't need an adjustable bench, or even a lot of sets to accomplish any of this. Just do walking push-ups. The Walking Push-up is an excellent total-chest and torso exercise. Due to the alternating arm position, you are forced to press from unusual angles, and the chest and delts are stimulated in a slightly different way than is experienced with the regular push-up. It also stresses the core, the waist, the front of the hips, and the legs — something bench pressing just can't do. Go slow, deep and strict for two painful sets.

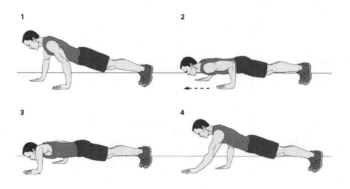

Walking Push-Up

Try — Horizontal Pull instead of Barbell Row.

No matter how many pull-ups you perform, to develop your upper back muscles to their full potential, you must perform horizontal pulling. Bending over and trying to maintain your position while holding a heavy bar is an accident waiting to happen. Horizontal rowing forces the upper back into new levels of strength and growth and develops a vice-like grip. Bodyweight variations will increase your athletic ability without screwing up your lower back.

Try — Squatting Calf Raises instead of Machine Calf Raise.

Because the calves carry your entire weight around all day, they are dense, powerful little muscles. This means that when you work your calves hard in the gym, you can build up to tremendous weights on the standing calf raise machine. You'll notice that the bodyweight squatting calf raise is harder than a regular calf raise. Why? The larger muscles of the calf (the gastrocnemius) cross the ankle, as well as the knee. The smaller calf muscle (called the soleus) only crosses the ankle. This means that when you bend your knees acutely, the larger calf muscles switch off, but the smaller muscles — those key to ankle strength and stability — are forced to do all the work.

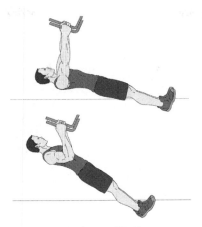

Horizontal Pull

Try — Hanging Grip Work and Rope Climbing instead of Wrist & Barbell Curls.

Curls are fun because they're easy, and they're easy because they only work the biceps. When you can get strong enough to climb rope without using your legs, it will give you huge biceps. Try climbing for two minutes going up, two going down, and you will develop a grip so strong that you'll fell like you can tear apart steel chains.

If you really want to build strong hands and forearms, you have to work your hands the way they evolved to work. Instead of a few puny sets of wrist curls and reverse wrist curls that wear down your wrists and provide little in the way of true lower arm strength and mass, follow a plan that will give you the strength to tear through phonebooks. There are plenty of ways to progress in hanging grip work, focus on time-based workouts. Try to extend the time you can hang each and every time you work out. When two arms are easy, move to one arm. Make sure you do your hanging work at the end of your routine or your pull-ups and hanging midsection work will suffer.

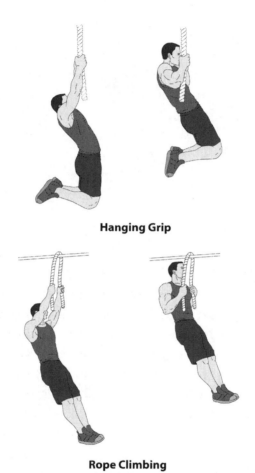

Hanging Grip

Rope Climbing

Try — Unilateral Triceps Dips instead of Skull-Crusher.

Lying triceps extensions are elbow wreckers because they stimulate the muscles without properly strengthening the axis joint, the elbow. Instead, try an exercise that will build total triceps mass and power while at the same time strengthening the all-important tendons of the wrist, forearm and elbow.

Unilateral triceps dips are tricky because they require balance, control and training intelligence. You can moderate the difficulty by altering your stance and get an elite level triceps workout anywhere.

[Bonus Resource – Unilateral tricep dip]

Try — Straight Bridges instead of Leg Curl.

Bridges will train your hamstrings while building a healthy spine and improving total body strength and flexibility. Bodybuilders and strength athletes who don't work bridges are missing out, and bridges are not just for wrestlers or Yoga weirdos.

[Bonus Resource – Straight Bridges effecting hamstrings]

Try — Tuck Jumps instead of Squats.

The Squat is viewed as the Holy Grail of exercises, but no one will deny that barbell squats can put a lot of stress on your spine.

No matter how serious you are about squatting, everyone takes a layoff from time to time, and maybe it's time to offset some nagging aches and pains. Tuck Jumps pack the legs and hips with speed, strength, and mass. Heavy barbell squatting is inevitably a fairly slow activity, and moving slowly all the time can de-train the nervous system. Why would your body be "explosive" if you never really move fast? Tuck jumps also work the hips and abs, training the legs to function as part of the anterior chain as well as a wonderful calf workout.

To do a tuck jump, start with a moderate, symmetrical stance, and explode up, tucking your knees as high into your chest as you can. When you land, don't pause, but use the momentum to dip immediately back down and spring up for rep two. Repeat. Build to three sets of twenty tuck jumps three times per week and you'll also get a cardio blast on top.

[Bonus Resource – Tuck Jump]

Try — Knee Squats instead of Weighted Lunges.

Instead of using lunges as a way to smoke your exhausted quads after a leg workout, use these as a finisher to re-balance any strength differential in the quadriceps. Various rep set and rep ranges can be applied, depending on where you place knee squats in your program.

An athlete who can manage fifty controlled reps on both legs is doing something right.

[Bonus Resource – Knee Squat or Shrimp]

Try — Human Flag instead of Weighted Side Bend.

Everyone knows how to work their abs, but when it comes to the obliques, people often just thrown a few side crunches or dumbbell side bends in as an afterthought. Likely it gets nothing at all. You don't need weights or crunches, performing a human flag will give you a waist like tempered steel, it will also work the hell out your grip, your arms, your shoulders, and your lats. The flag requires you to be really strong in every muscle of your body and will reveal your weak links quickly.

[Bonus Resource – Human Flag]

Try — Rollovers instead of the Cardio Rowing Machine.

The rowing machine develops pulling strength, works the entire body as a unit, and develops stamina and lung power. However, you can get a full body cardio workout plus pulling power, grip strength, and a hardcore waist workout with rollovers.

Jump up and hang from a high bar with a shoulder-width grip. Lift your feet as you pull down, and lever your legs right up and around over the bar. Let your body follow your feet, and control your descent until you are hanging back where you started. That's one rep. Simply roll yourself up and around the bar, right back to where you started. It's tricky at first, but you soon get into a rhythm.

Once you can do fifty rollovers in a row, your total body cardio power will be through the roof.

[Bonus Resource – Rollover]

Work toward mastering the Big Six, and fit them into your normal training. I've given you a strategy for mastering them, and listed below are the elite strength standards for the more advanced "Perfect 10."

1. Pistol squat: 25 reps per leg. Requires hip, knee and ankle

strength, mobility and endurance. Tree trunk legs, guaranteed.

2. Push-up: 100 reps. Requires pressing strength and stamina. Shirt popping chest, guaranteed.
3. Pull-up: 50 reps. Requires an iron grip, pulling strength and stamina. Pop-eye forearms and barn door lats, guaranteed.
4. Muscle-up: 10 reps. Requires explosive athleticism involving both pulling and pushing strength. Upper body thickness, guaranteed.
5. Elbow lever: 1-minute hold. Requires isometric balance, strength, and stamina. Horse-shoe triceps guaranteed.
6. Human Flag: 5 seconds. Requires total lateral chain power. The world record is 15 seconds. Three-dimensional obliques and shoulders, guaranteed.
7. Front lever: 10 seconds. Requires total-body coordination with an emphasis on anterior chain strength. Injury proof back, guaranteed.
8. Back lever: 10 seconds. The opposite direction of the front lever, requiring more flexibility and plenty of posterior chain strength.
9. L-Sit hold: 20 seconds. Requires hip flexibility and total abdominal power. Visible abs that look like a stack of bricks, guaranteed.
10. Free handstand: 30 seconds: Requires shoulder and arm strength, balance, and a solid core. Ninja status to all bystanders, guaranteed.

As you can see, the possibilities are endless and the chains of gym membership are released. I wish you good luck and longevity in the pursuit of muscle and strength. Eat right, sleep well, train hard, and you will unlock your full potential. No one was born "strong" and it's about the adventure, not the destination. Appreciate the process, and allow fitness to contribute to the quality of your life instead of being the focus of it. A positive mental attitude and dedication toward the mastery of any skill will allow you to reap its rewards in many aspects of your life.

Self-mastery is the most noble pursuit of them all. Habits and skills can all be trained. Develop a growth mind-set and cultivate mindfulness to enjoy life to the fullest. These techniques give you control over your emotional state in any situation and serve you on your journey to excellence. Embrace the pain of weakness leaving your body and recognize that you must fail in order to get stronger at anything.

You can do it. The power of better habits starts now!

Ready to Live a High Intensity Life?

If you're someone who struggles with your weight, sticking to a training regimen, and you've tried just about everything… you're not alone. Whether you're almost ready to give up, or if you're can't seem to get the results you've been promised from all the fancy training methods, pills, potions and powders, by picking up this book, you're clearly willing to give it one more shot.

Ignoring your lack of progress, and continuing to swing a hammer of stubbornness and tenacity at the same nail will only frustrate you further. Never try to change your results by fighting with your existing reality. In order to truly change something, you have to use a new system that makes the old system obsolete.

Maybe you're a busy executive who is more interested in having limitless energy when in challenging client meetings, than sculpting your guns with moronic meatheads. You might be trying to get back into shape, or you're already fit, but you know you could do better. Change is inevitable, but growth is a personal choice.

You believe that it's important to continuously challenge yourself, physically as well as mentally, for continued development, but you've had a hard time finding a program that delivers HALF of what it promises. Which, in reality, is really just recycled information that doesn't work all that well to begin with.

If you're like me, you've spent thousands on supplements, training programs, and maybe even hired a personal trainer only to be disappointed again and again. Stop wasting tons of money, but worse that that - TIME.

You know you have to commit to a routine in order to get results. You do this to be a more effective leader, and let's be honest… to look good naked.

Not committing to the right regimen will leave you tired, frustrated, and maybe even worse -injured and sick! Unhealthier still, would be not doing anything at all. That will leave you weak, mentally, leading to depression or Alzheimer's.

Physically, we know that 65% of Americans are overweight which contributes to the number one killer in the United States: Heart Disease! You will not live a healthy life without going about your days intentionally.

You can't close your eyes and make it go away. You will not age gracefully without a practice of strength training for your mind and body, but you're not sold on the idea of yoga class.

I know how you feel. There is so much confusion out there. Ignorance is the root of all our problems, and complexity is the enemy of action. I spent 10 years struggling to make progress, and I finally figured it out once I was forced to quit.

You see, I became an executive in the construction industry and I was forced to work long hours as well as travel to hotels all over the country. I was committed though. I would drive to the gym no matter the traffic or distance. I skipped social events in order to dedicate time to bench, squat, and deadlift. And for what?

When my life was in complete disarray and I drew that final straw, I quit everything.

I was 30 years old, and I saw my entire life flash before my eyes... my 20s flew by, and I realized I was climbing the wrong corporate ladder. I put in my two-week notification, sold everything I owned, and drove West.

Needless to say, a $200 gym membership wasn't in the cards, but I always knew there was another way to implement a training system to make strength a priority. I researched old gymnastic books, read all of the Convict Conditioning E-Books, and studied under some awesome meditation and breathing gurus.

Hundreds of hours spent reading, experimenting, and training while I was on the road trying to find my own path, lead me to the conclusion: You need to get everything you can, out of what you have before you ever set foot in a gym.

Can you do 10 handstand pushups?

I could Military Press 195, but I couldn't.

How about decline-one-arm pushups?

I could bench 345, but I couldn't.

20 Pistol squats? One-arm pull-ups?

Nope.

How about hold your breath for 4 minutes? Take a 20-minute ice bath?

No way.

There are all kinds of personal challenges you can do without paying for a coach or membership. If you can't perform these body-weight feats of strength first, why are you paying anyone anything?

Look at the bodies of gymnasts, from the high school level all the way to the Olympic level. Their level of musculature is incredible. I'll let you in on a secret - they don't train with barbells or "sculpt their guns."

Better yet, look at the physiques of the ancient Greek statues. Those bodies were developed before there were cameras, Photoshop, steroids, or cable machines! They developed their muscles with progressive bodyweight exercises, not with modern bodybuilding techniques.

I was big and "strong" after 10-years in the gym, but I was soft, sick, and didn't look the part at all. I certainly didn't look like the fitness models on magazine covers. In reality, I was embarrassed to take my shirt off despite all of my training efforts.

There is an easier and healthier way to build a body that will serve you, long after the bro's at big-box gyms give up on their relentless pursuit of the pump. Trust me, I know. I was one of them.

I took the best of the methods I learned lifting in the gym, combined it with the advice I got from bodyweight training experts, and I FINALLY started getting results.

To make some money while I was on the road, I started training people to get the same. I found out that I wasn't the only one who struggled with this information. So many people were benefiting from my insights that I wrote them all down.

This book will guide you through the steps to get you where you want to be. No matter what strength level you're at or where you are in the world: you can perform this routine.

If you're not getting the results you want from your current program, I'm excited that you're going to give mine a try. I've got license to brag because I didn't make any of this stuff up. I've simply compiled the best training I've gathered "in the trenches," books, seminars, and great teachers from all over the world.

Just ask any one of my now shredded clients who are pound-for-pound now some of the strongest people I've seen.

Imagine being able to cancel your gym membership in order to make more progress at home, or simply adding some of these training principles to your current split. Trust me, you're going to want to reconsider how much time and money you're spending once you see what's really possible.

Imagine what it would feel like to continue to hone your mental clarity so that you're able to crush it in business and in relationships. You now have the tools to finally get results that stick.

I want you to make sure you reach out to me online at **www. highintensitylife.com** if you have any comments, questions, or concerns about any of the material in this book. Better yet, reach out if you're ready to know what the next step is. There you'll find my free 5-minute Spartan Meditation Guide, workbooks, and further support.

Lucky for you, people have been getting strong and muscular using their own bodyweight for thousands of years. This program works. If you don't already know the power of meditation, when you incorporate it with these training methods, you'll be able to go deeper into your mind and physiology that you ever thought possible. Make sure you follow up online.

You can have the results you seek. If any of this material resonates with you, do not hesitate to get after your goals or reach out to me for support. Excellence is simply a commitment to completion, and all that must be asked is, "Am I willing to do it?".

Everything in this world is built twice. First in your imagination, second with your next actions. Become an observer of your own thoughts.

If you're someone who struggles to focus on one course until successful, and you get easily distracted. Maybe you suffer from indecision, or are feeling anxiety about where you are versus where you know you should be. You continue to mull over the best course of action, and worry that you don't have enough information to make the right decisions...

Ignoring this problem will only make things worse. Anxiety and stress have been known literally kill you, and indecision is the death of Great men.

It's impossible to avoid pain and mental discomfort, but our suffering comes from our reaction to it. Physical discomfort is unavoidable, but we make things worse than than they need to be. Listen to your thoughts, but understand that they do not define you or the situation.

Your fear isn't you.

Your anxiety isn't you.

Experiencing fear does not make you a coward. The real you is merely aware of the role these thoughts and feelings play. Being mindful is not a matter of thinking more clearly about an experience; it is the act of experiencing life with clarity.

Meditation is a tool to help increase your awareness and focus, which allows you to see that your thoughts are just passing impressions. It develops the mind's ability to see things the way they really are.

Becoming an observer of your thoughts and worries will allow you to overcome their power over you. I know how you feel because I've been there! I found a simple little trick that showed me the way out.

Developing an immense capacity for sustained concentration is something anyone can do, anywhere. It's the WILL that you learn to concentrate with.

The will, to the mind, would be like a magnifying glass with the sun. It focuses your energy and brings it zeroing in on one spot.

Focusing on the now is the key to taking the best action, eliminating anxiety, and achieving happiness. Seeking pleasures and avoiding pain will not result in happiness because our pleasures are fleeting. Even if you achieve the ultimate moment of pleasure - pure bliss. Your feelings will fade, and you'll move on to chasing the next moment.

Meditation has been practiced all over the world by high-performers for thousands of years, and concentration is how you move mountains.

Napoleon Bonaparte said, "I see only the objective, the obstacle must give way."

Concentration is the key to your success, and it's built through meditation.

...But I wasn't willing to commit to the massive costs of Transcendental Meditation or the time commitment of an hour long Yoga class.

Imagine what it will feel like when you're no longer chasing fleeting feelings or looking no further than what's directly in front of you. Our decisions are often based on perceptions rather than reality. Meditation gives you the ability to control your emotional state so that you can look at things in a different way.

There is more to living life and finding happiness than merely seeking pleasure and avoiding pain. This is clear for the warriors who seek to overcome adversity, put pleasure aside, and to walk calmly through the fire.

We must strengthen our will, and know that the process will require some dedication. It does not, however, require a massive amount of time.

If we seek to master our mind, we must bolster our brain power in the same way we train the body. Iron sharpens iron, as one man sharpens another. Train your mind, or you know what they say, "Use it or loose it." No more weak mental muscles.

I encourage you in this book to develop a mediation habit, but I go deeper online, where I've created a free report. You'll learn the simple little trick that makes meditation easy, doable, and painless. Anyone can do it.

You'll also get a guide for Spartan thinking so you can focus on what really matters: objectives and results. Laid out are proven, repeatable, methods that will develop your iron will, anywhere, in five minutes a day. Train quietly in your own "Mind-Gym" with a combat-hardened veteran not some guru with expensive magic dust.

It's free, so make sure you download it, and keep in touch!

www.HighIntensityLife.com

57456746R00076

Made in the USA
Lexington, KY
14 November 2016